NEW DIRECTIONS FOR EVALUATION
A PUBLICATION OF THE AMERICAN EVALUATION ASSOCIATION

Gary T. Henry, *Georgia State University*
COEDITOR-IN-CHIEF

Jennifer C. Greene, *University of Illinois*
COEDITOR-IN-CHIEF

Conducting Multiple Site Evaluations in Real-World Settings

James M. Herrell
Center for Substance Abuse Treatment/Substance Abuse and Mental Health Services Administration

Roger B. Straw
Health Resources and Services Administration

EDITORS

Number 94, Summer 2002

JOSSEY-BASS
San Francisco

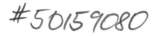

CONDUCTING MULTIPLE SITE EVALUATIONS IN REAL-WORLD SETTINGS
James M. Herrell, Roger B. Straw (eds.)
New Directions for Evaluation, no. 94
Jennifer C. Greene, Gary T. Henry, Coeditors-in-Chief
Copyright ©2002 Wiley Periodicals, Inc., A Wiley Company

Microfilm copies of issues and articles are available in 16mm and 35mm, as well as microfiche in 105mm, through University Microfilms Inc., 300 North Zeeb Road, Ann Arbor, Michigan 48106-1346.

New Directions for Evaluation is indexed in Contents Pages in Education, Higher Education Abstracts, and Sociological Abstracts.

Print ISSN: 1097-6736; Online ISSN: 1534-875X ISBN: 0-7879-6345-3

NEW DIRECTIONS FOR EVALUATION is part of The Jossey-Bass Education Series and is published quarterly by Wiley Subscription Services, Inc., A Wiley Company, at Jossey-Bass, 989 Market Street, San Francisco, California 94103-1741.

SUBSCRIPTIONS cost $69.00 for U.S./Canada/Mexico; $93 international. For institutions, agencies, and libraries, $145 U.S.; $185 Canada; $219 international. Prices subject to change.

EDITORIAL CORRESPONDENCE should be addressed to the Editors-in-Chief, Jennifer C. Greene, Department of Educational Psychology, University of Illinois, 260E Education Building, 1310 South Sixth Street, Champaign, IL 61820, or Gary T. Henry, School of Policy Studies, Georgia State University, P.O. Box 4039, Atlanta, GA 30302-4039.

www.josseybass.com

Printed in the United States of America on acid-free recycled paper containing at least 20 percent postconsumer waste.

New Directions for Evaluation

Sponsored by the American Evaluation Association

Editorial Policy and Procedures

New Directions for Evaluation, a quarterly sourcebook, is an official publication of the American Evaluation Association. The journal publishes empirical, methodological, and theoretical works on all aspects of evaluation. A reflective approach to evaluation is an essential strand to be woven through every volume. The editors encourage volumes that have one of three foci: (1) craft volumes that present approaches, methods, or techniques that can be applied in evaluation practice, such as the use of templates, case studies, or survey research; (2) professional issue volumes that present issues of import for the field of evaluation, such as utilization of evaluation or locus of evaluation capacity; (3) societal issue volumes that draw out the implications of intellectual, social, or cultural developments for the field of evaluation, such as the women's movement, communitarianism, or multiculturalism. A wide range of substantive domains is appropriate for *New Directions for Evaluation;* however, the domains must be of interest to a large audience within the field of evaluation. We encourage a diversity of perspectives and experiences within each volume, as well as creative bridges between evaluation and other sectors of our collective lives.

The editors do not consider or publish unsolicited single manuscripts. Each issue of the journal is devoted to a single topic, with contributions solicited, organized, reviewed, and edited by a guest editor. Issues may take any of several forms, such as a series of related chapters, a debate, or a long article followed by brief critical commentaries. In all cases, the proposals must follow a specific format, which can be obtained from the editor-in-chief. These proposals are sent to members of the editorial board and to relevant substantive experts for peer review. The process may result in acceptance, a recommendation to revise and resubmit, or rejection. However, the editors are committed to working constructively with potential guest editors to help them develop acceptable proposals.

Jennifer C. Greene, Coeditor-in-Chief
Department of Educational Psychology
University of Illinois
260E Education Building
1310 South Sixth Street
Champaign, IL 61820
e-mail:jcgreene@uiuc.edu

Gary T. Henry, Coeditor-in-Chief
School of Policy Studies
Georgia State University
P.O. Box 4039
Atlanta, GA 30302-4039
e-mail: gthenry@gsu.edu

CONTENTS

EDITORS' NOTES

In 1991, Sinacore and Turpin coined the term *multisite evaluation* to describe what they observed to be a relatively common type of evaluation that had not received much attention in the evaluation literature (Turpin and Sinacore, 1991). During the decade since Sinacore and Turpin's volume in the *New Directions for Evaluation* series, interest in multisite evaluations has grown, with a nascent body of literature on the issues involved in conducting evaluations in multiple sites. For instance, the literature on clinical trials increasingly contains references to the issues that arise in conducting multicenter clinical trials (Friedman, Furberg, and DeMets, 1998; Murray, 1998).

Our purpose in this volume is to derive lessons about the design, implementation, and value of multisite evaluations from five programs initiated during the past decade by the Substance Abuse and Mental Health Services Administration (SAMHSA). In particular, we emphasize the importance of phase of research and departure from the gold standard for multisite clinical trials in the design and conduct of multisite evaluations and the analysis and interpretation of data. Although all studies described in this volume were funded by a single agency (SAMHSA) and examine the impact of interventions on persons with mental illness or substance abuse disorders, we seek to develop lessons for the evaluation field in general.

We selected programs and evaluations that vary along key dimensions. Some studies are more exploratory, others confirmatory. One is a multicenter randomized clinical trial, with common interventions, measures, and other standardization across sites. Others vary markedly along important study characteristics, such as the consistency across sites of the interventions being studied. Some of the studies were implemented to determine whether anything worked; others were intended to define the relative effectiveness of programs already shown to be efficacious. The five programs also share significant commonalities, reflecting the realities of federally funded multisite evaluations in the mental health and substance abuse fields. Four of the programs evaluated actual interventions as practiced in the field, and the fifth (examined in Chapter Two), although a true multisite clinical trial, evaluated treatments based on validated approaches delivered by experienced therapists to a diverse set of clients in community-based settings.

In each case, the persons responsible for conceptualizing, implementing, and evaluating the interventions were the same; SAMHSA's grant announcements called for the grantees to develop, deliver, and evaluate the interventions, in conjunction with SAMHSA staff. Although external evaluators may often attempt to build teams and steering committees such as those described in this volume, the level of coordination and collaboration within and across sites and the degree to which the federal funding agency had an active role are consistently high in the programs selected here. Furthermore, consistent with the mission of SAMHSA during the period these programs were funded, the primary purpose of the programs was to generate new and useful knowledge that would directly affect policy and practice.

Collectively, these five programs represent a number of challenges in evaluation planning, management, and implementation; study design; and data-analytic approaches. Although the studies described in this volume represent an approach to multisite evaluation that has much in common with the clinical trials tradition, they share with cluster evaluation an appreciation for the adjustments that are necessary to reflect the realities of conducting evaluation research in real-world service settings.

Chapter One briefly describes the range of evaluation activities characterized as multisite evaluations and presents a framework for addressing important issues in planning and conducting multisite evaluations. Chapters Two through Six discuss evaluation and its challenges associated with five SAMHSA-sponsored multisite studies. In the final chapter, two evaluators who have been involved in a number of multisite evaluations interpret the other chapters in view of their own experiences and the questions posed in Chapter One.

In Chapter One, Straw and Herrell discuss definitional and conceptual issues related to multiple site evaluation studies, present a conceptual framework for understanding such studies, and pose questions for determining the appropriateness of particular types of multiple site evaluations for specific purposes.

Babor, Steinberg, McRee, Vendetti, and Carroll discuss in Chapter Two the Marijuana Treatment Project, funded by the Center for Substance Abuse Treatment (CSAT) in 1996. This project examined the clinical efficacy of two brief treatments for chronic marijuana abuse by adults. The study, a randomized multisite clinical trial, was selected for discussion in this volume to demonstrate the feasibility of conducting rigorous multisite clinical trials in field settings and to examine factors contributing to the success of such trials.

The Employment Intervention Demonstration Program, funded in 1995 by the Center for Mental Health Services (CMHS), was the first SAMHSA multisite evaluation study to require the use of a common data collection protocol that was developed collaboratively by the participating sites. Cook, Carey, Razzano, Burke, and Blyler discuss in Chapter Three the influence of the phase of research on the development of the program, the role of participants and stakeholders in shaping the common protocol, the dissemination of early findings, and the impact of the program on policy.

The Collaborative Program to Prevent Homelessness, jointly funded in 1996 by CMHS and CSAT and examined in Chapter Four, illustrates a multisite study designed to explore the relative effectiveness of several interventions developed to ameliorate homelessness among persons with mental illness and substance abuse disorders. Banks, McHugo, Williams, Drake, and Shinn describe an innovative, prospective meta-analytic approach to the analysis of multisite data when cross-site variation does not allow for the pooling of data.

The CMHS Housing Initiative, explored in Chapter Five, illustrates a multisite study that explicitly planned to build on the existing knowledge base on supported housing for individuals with serious mental illnesses. Rog and Randolph describe how the readiness for study of a supported housing intervention model affected the development of a multisite evaluation; they also describe the advantages of conducting a multisite study even when there are barriers to implementation.

Initiated in 1998 by CSAT, the Methamphetamine Treatment Project is a multisite study intended to evaluate whether a manualized substance abuse intervention (that is, implemented in accordance with a well-defined written protocol) shown to be effective for a particular drug (cocaine) would also be effective for a different drug (methamphetamine). In Chapter Six, Rawson, Marinelli-Casey, and Huber discuss the design and management of a multisite comparison of one standard intervention against seven site-specific, treatment-as-usual interventions.

Drawing on their experience as evaluators of several multiple site studies, Leff and Mulkern in Chapter Seven interpret the other chapters and derive lessons for multisite evaluations. They emphasize the important and sometimes competing contributions to multisite evaluations of the methods of science and the needs of stakeholders, and they offer guidelines for conducting the most valuable multisite evaluations given the phase of research, the constraints of conducting evaluations in real-world settings, and the needs of the treatment field, the funding agencies, and stakeholders.

James M. Herrell
Roger B. Straw
Editors

References

Friedman, L. M., Furberg, C. D., and DeMets, D. L. *Fundamentals of Clinical Trials*. (3rd ed.) New York: Springer-Verlag, 1998.

Murray, D. M. "Design and Analysis of Group-Randomized Trials." *Monographs in Epidemiology and Biostatistics*, 1998, 27 (entire issue).

Turpin, R. S., and Sinacore, J. M. (Eds.). *Multisite Evaluations*. New Directions for Evaluation, no. 50. San Francisco: Jossey-Bass, 1991.

JAMES M. HERRELL is a social science analyst with the Center for Substance Abuse Treatment, Substance Abuse and Mental Health Services Administration, U.S. Department of Health and Human Services.

ROGER B. STRAW is director of the Division of Planning and Evaluation, Office of Planning and Evaluation, Health Resources and Services Administration, U.S. Department of Health and Human Services.

1

Multisite evaluations are increasingly being used by the federal government and large foundations. A framework for understanding the variations among multisite evaluations and developing ways to improve them is presented in this chapter.

A Framework for Understanding and Improving Multisite Evaluations

Roger B. Straw, James M. Herrell

Turpin and Sinacore (1991) were among the first authors to use the term *multisite evaluation* (MSE) and to note the unique demands of evaluating programs at different geographical locations. They pointed out that there were no accepted criteria for defining an MSE and no literature that explicitly addressed the issues intrinsic to these evaluations. They distinguished between MSEs examining interventions that are implemented in the same way across all sites and those that examined different interventions or variations of the same intervention across sites. In the subsequent decade, there has been growing interest in, and publication of articles related to, MSE, but there are still no accepted criteria for defining MSEs, no accepted terminology for distinguishing among such evaluations, and no general guidelines for determining the most appropriate type of MSE for a given purpose.

This chapter provides a brief descriptive overview of the range of evaluation activities that have been characterized as MSEs. It then presents a framework for addressing important issues in planning and conducting a particular subtype of MSE that has much in common with multicenter clinical trials.

What Is a Multisite Evaluation?

Although Sinacore and Turpin (1991) did not offer an explicit definition of MSE, it is implicit in their presentation that two factors differentiate MSEs from other evaluation activities: the involvement of multiple sites and the conduct of a cross-site evaluation activity. The number of sites can vary from two or three to fifty or more. What constitutes a site can also vary considerably.

NEW DIRECTIONS FOR EVALUATION, no. 94, Summer 2002   © Wiley Periodicals, Inc.

For example, an MSE could involve comparisons among individual classrooms in a school (as learning environments, for instance). It could also involve, as it does in all of the chapters in this volume, distinct geographical locations where some programmatic intervention, such as substance abuse or mental health treatment, is being studied. Finally, the intervention being studied may be required to be the same in each site or be allowed to vary across sites.

The nature of the cross-site evaluation activity can also vary. It can be retrospective (relying on data already collected by the sites) or prospective (the cross-site evaluator is involved in the data collection process). The purpose of the evaluation can range from providing information for program improvement (more formative purposes) to generating estimates of the efficacy and effectiveness of a specific intervention strategy (more summative purposes).

These and other important factors distinguish MSEs from other evaluation activities. MSEs may be longer (for example, three to five years) and cost more (for example, several million dollars) than single-site evaluations. MSEs may often involve a coordinated cross-site study, with each participating site providing data to a centrally managed evaluation, as well as conducting local project-specific evaluation activities, further adding to the cost. In part because of the their cost and scope, MSE initiatives typically are funded by government organizations or by large foundations with explicit interests in developing knowledge that will be relevant to broad policy-oriented audiences and can be used to change practice.

Although frequently not acknowledged as such, many evaluations (and particularly federally funded evaluations) are MSEs. For example, a number of the landmark studies in the early years of evaluation were, in fact, MSEs. The New Jersey Negative Income Tax Experiment (Kershaw and Fair, 1976) involved the random assignment of thirteen hundred families in four New Jersey communities and one Pennsylvania community to eight different conditions. The RAND Health Insurance Experiment (Newhouse and others, 1981) involved twenty-seven hundred families in six communities. Randomized clinical trials often employ multiple sites to enroll patients more quickly into protocols. Many prevention and education evaluations are conducted in multiple communities, schools, or classrooms; such studies are, by their nature, MSE studies.

Why Conduct Multisite Evaluations?

There are a number of important reasons to consider conducting an MSE. The most obvious is the inability to obtain an adequate sample in an individual site. One might need multiple sites to increase overall sample size for statistical power or to obtain the needed sample size more quickly. Similarly, multiple sites might be required in order to obtain an adequate sample in particular population subgroups (for example, minorities or particular age cohorts). Furthermore, there may be an interest in examining the impact of a particular intervention across a range of geographical locations (or, more generically, a range of contexts).

There are additional reasons cited in the literature for sponsoring MSE studies. For example, reasons for which the W. K. Kellogg Foundation funds MSEs include accumulating knowledge more rapidly, increasing the policy impact of a particular funding initiative, and increasing the amount or rate of systemic change. MSE studies can provide opportunities for evaluators and other stakeholders to work together on difficult issues and to identify intervention and contextual factors that affect the impact of interventions (Worthen and Schmitz, 1997). Finally, some organizations include building evaluation capacity in local communities among their purposes in conducting an MSE.

Are There Different Types of Multisite Evaluation?

In the past few years, three relatively distinct types of evaluations that involve multiple sites have become evident: cluster evaluations, multisite (sometimes called cross-site) evaluations, and multicenter clinical trials. Table 1.1 summarizes some of the important differences among the types of MSE. The table is reasonably self-explanatory, except for the final dimension: model of cross-site evaluation. By a collaborative model of cross-site evaluation, we mean that although there may be a lead evaluator (for instance, a coordinating center), the lead cross-site evaluator must establish and maintain a collaborative relationship with the sites to develop and implement a successful MSE. By a national model of cross-site evaluation, we mean that the funding source may dictate the evaluation model or may vest fuller authority in the cross-site evaluator to lead the evaluation and will expect sites to follow the lead. In either model, collaboration and goodwill are necessary for a successful evaluation.

Cluster evaluations (see, for example, Barley and Jenness, 1993, and Worthen and Schmitz, 1997) are most often associated with the W. K. Kellogg Foundation, which developed the idea and has funded many of the existing cluster evaluations. Cluster evaluations are often associated with Kellogg Foundation initiatives that encourage local communities to develop partnerships that will result in significant systems change within the community. As used by the Kellogg Foundation, cluster evaluation examines initiatives or interventions based in local communities to identify common themes or components that are associated with positive impacts, as well as the reasons for these associations. Cluster evaluators are expected to maintain collaborative relationships with both local projects and the foundation's program staff. Information obtained from the individual projects is confidential

Table 1.1. Variation Across Types of Multisite Evaluation on Important Dimensions

Dimension	Cluster Evaluation	Multisite Evaluation	Multicenter Clinical Trial
Principal purpose	Examine variation	Estimate impact or examine variation	Estimate impact
Phase of research	Exploratory	Exploratory to confirmatory	Confirmatory
Source of intervention	Program driven	Program, early data driven	Research driven
Standardization	Extensive variation	Some to extensive variation	Extensive standardization
Timing of cross-site evaluation	Planned to retrospective	Planned to retrospective	Planned
Role of cross-site evaluation	Formative	Summative	Summative
Model of cross-site evaluation	Collaborative	National evaluator to collaborative	Collaborative

and reported to the Kellogg Foundation only in aggregate form. Cluster evaluators are expected to assemble evidence about whether the foundation program efforts contributed to their desired ends but are explicitly not expected to provide rigorous estimates of effectiveness. Cluster evaluators are also expected to work with the individual sites and to share their observations (that is, to adopt a formative evaluation stance).

MSEs are frequently associated with federally funded programs (including demonstration programs). This type of evaluation is often dependent on the data collected by the individual sites and may often impose a national evaluation on sites that have been in operation for some time. The evaluations typically involve variation across sites—sometimes considerable—in interventions or measurements, although there is often an effort to develop a core set of measures used in all sites. The common measures are used to estimate the effectiveness of the interventions and examine variation across sites in outcomes (a more summative evaluation focus than is involved with cluster evaluation). Cook and others (Chapter Three, this volume) describe a variation of this approach that involves both a coordinated multicenter evaluation and a series of site-specific studies, which those authors refer to as a multisite-plus-stand-alone study design. In recent years, the Substance Abuse and Mental Health Services Administration (SAMHSA), as well as a number of other organizations, sought to overcome some of the problems associated with these evaluations by reducing the types and amounts of variations across sites, including on occasion the use of multicenter clinical trials.

Multicenter clinical trials (see, for example, Friedman, Furberg, and DeMets, 1998, and Meinert, 1986) are randomized (or Phase III) clinical trials that are conducted in multiple sites for the primary purposes of increasing sample size, improving the representativeness of the study population, or ensuring that the intervention is efficacious in multiple settings (or contexts). The emphasis in multicenter clinical trials is on reducing variation across sites in the sampled population, intervention, measurements, and evaluation procedures. The very tight control over all aspects of the study separates the multicenter clinical trial from the other types of MSEs. However, the literature on multicenter clinical trials increasingly acknowledges the need to include measures to identify variations across sites in the delivery and receipt of the intervention, as well as potential differences in clinic settings that could affect outcomes (see, for example, Kraemer, 2000).

Although many studies that have contributed substantially to our knowledge of the effectiveness of interventions for mental illness and substance abuse disorders are MSEs, attention is often not given within these studies to multisite issues. For instance, Jainchill, Hawke, De Leon, and Yagelka (2000) conducted a multisite study of outcomes for adolescents receiving substance abuse treatment in therapeutic communities. Data were gathered on adolescent admissions to six treatment sites. Data were pooled for analysis, program variation was not reported, and logistic regression was used to establish predictors of outcomes. Furthermore, consumers and reviewers of these studies may ignore the contributions and problems attributable to involving multiple sites. Williams, Chang, and the Addiction Centre Adolescent Research Group (2000), for instance, reviewed findings from eight major multisite studies of the treatment of adolescent substance abuse, but in their discussion of methodological issues, they did not mention the degree of attention within the studies to multisite issues.

Multisite Evaluation in SAMHSA

Over the past decade, SAMHSA has funded increasingly complex and structured program evaluations intended to develop improved interventions for individuals with mental illness and substance abuse disorders and to transfer those interventions into treatment programs across the country. In the early years, these efforts were typically characterized as demonstration programs (Straw, Levine, and Osher, 1997). The evaluations were based on a simple phased approach that began with problem identification through epidemiological and descriptive research. Once the basic parameters of the problem were known, MSEs were funded to examine either research-based or existing programs designed to ameliorate the problems or to develop new programs and explore their effectiveness. On the basis of these exploratory studies, rigorous tests of the programs with preliminary evidence of effectiveness would be conducted. Finally, the programs with confirmed effectiveness could be systematically documented and disseminated to the field as proven models for adoption within community service programs. These "replicated" programs could be studied to examine whether the adaptations changed the level of effectiveness. In the mid-1990s, SAMHSA adapted this approach to knowledge development into its current Knowledge Development and Application strategy for improving the effectiveness of community-based programs for the prevention and treatment of mental illness and substance abuse disorders.

SAMHSA has supported numerous evaluations that range along the full continuum of MSEs. For instance, Tinsman and others (2001) report findings from a cross-site study of twelve outreach projects for human immunodeficiency virus, sponsored by the Center for Substance Abuse Treatment. This cross-site study was developed after the projects were funded and in operation; a common set of data elements was developed through a data coordinating center, with all sites contributing. Otherwise, there was little standardization across sites, with each grantee defining its own target population and developing its intervention. At the opposite end of the spectrum of MSEs supported by SAMHSA is a multicenter clinical trial of brief treatments for marijuana dependence (see Chapter Two, this volume).

A Multisite Evaluation Framework

No approach to categorizing MSEs has gained general acceptance. Hanrahan and others (1999) and Springer (2000) have suggested *multiple site evaluation* as a generic term for an evaluation in which two or more sites engage in a coordinated effort to address a core set of study questions. We propose adopting this term to describe the large multidimensional space associated with these types of evaluations. We propose the use of *cluster evaluation* for MSEs employing limited cross-site evaluations that are relatively formative or exploratory and involve relatively large site-to-site variation along key dimensions, such as the type of intervention being studied or target population. We will use *multicenter clinical trial* to refer to rigorous Phase III clinical trials involving more than one site that intend to employ identical interventions and evaluation procedures. Between these areas in the multidimensional space are MSEs, more rigorous and standardized than cluster evaluations but lacking the uniformity across sites that characterize a multicenter clinical trial.

To date, the process of planning and implementing cluster evaluations and MSEs has often been a relatively unstructured activity that depends heavily on the skills of the individuals involved in each study. Although the planning and implementation of multicenter clinical trials are more highly structured, issues associated with conducting clinical trials in multiple sites are often neglected (Kraemer, 2000). Because of the cost and time typically associated with conducting multiple site evaluations, a more systematic approach to deciding when, and how, to conduct a multiple site evaluation is needed.

The framework depicted in Table 1.1 is offered as a starting point for developing guidelines for the planners of these types of studies. The framework borrows heavily from a phases-of-research perspective (Flay, 1986; Holder and others, 1999). The source of interventions to be studied—that is, the extent to which the interventions derive from research or from programs as practiced—is likely to drive the planning and implementation of the studies. Research-based interventions will usually have a broader base of information that can be used in planning than will program-based interventions. Studies involving program-based interventions will probably need to spend more time and resources during the multiple site evaluation developing this base of information and therefore will have less ability to address effectiveness questions.

The phase of research may also be related to the degree of standardization required across sites and the resources devoted to rigorous estimates of effectiveness. Exploratory studies more often will need to focus on documenting the components of interventions and developing evidence supporting effectiveness with limited efforts to impose standardization across sites. Confirmatory studies (that is, multicenter clinical trials) ideally will be conducted only after exploratory studies have provided evidence of effectiveness and should focus resources on increased rigor of study design and measurement. Replication studies would focus on measuring the adaptations made by individual sites and the effects of those adaptations on the effectiveness of the previously tested intervention.

Challenges in Designing and Implementing Multiple Site Evaluations

The design and implementation of MSEs involve all of the challenges that are typically faced in designing any other evaluation study, as well as a few additional ones. Some would argue that the multicenter clinical trial is the gold standard for designing and implementing multiple site evaluations. The trial must be centrally coordinated, there must be a core set of study questions that all sites address, the target population must be clearly defined and applied across sites, measurement points and instruments must be standard across sites, and there must be a set of quality assurance procedures in place to promote consistency across therapists and others involved in the intervention, interviewers, and data recorders. Hanrahan and others (1999) proposed a continuum, with the multicenter clinical trial at one end and MSEs that depart significantly from the essential or defining ingredients of a clinical trial at the other. Springer (2000) proposed extending the continuum past MSEs to meta-analytic reviews. In these multiple site evaluations, the number of sites is too large or the variation across sites too great to permit data pooling for analytic purposes, so meta-analytic procedures are used.

Our belief is that multiple site evaluations that depart from the multicenter clinical trial ideal are not necessarily weaker or less appropriate studies. The multicenter clinical trial is most likely to be ideal when assessing the efficacy and effectiveness of well-specified (or research-driven) interventions in comparison to well-defined controls. We believe that this will rarely be the case in community settings. Therefore, in developing an appropriate evaluation design, one should consider the purpose of the evaluation, the principal questions, the phase of research, financial constraints, and feasibility of different designs (for example, whether randomization can be ethically or realistically employed). Dennis, Perl, Huebner, and McLellan (2000) note that although randomized studies are most appropriate for asking questions about the relative effectiveness or cost-effectiveness of different interventions, they may be totally inappropriate for other questions and may be no more effective than quasi-experiments for many purposes. They also argue that for many policy or programmatic issues, quasi-experimental designs are adequate for decision purposes. These authors encourage evaluators to match the research design to the question and to use hybrid designs: "Most treatment services research studies address multiple questions, work with heterogeneous populations, and thus should utilize a hybrid research design" (p. S287).

When an MSE is contemplated, a number of issues must be addressed. In many cases, the question is the extent to which all participating sites will be required to conform to a single decision. For example, will all sites be required to randomize individuals? Will all sites use the same inclusion and exclusion criteria?

Evaluation Questions. Is the primary evaluation question one that requires an MSE? For example, is there a need to study variations across settings or populations? Are multiple sites necessary to complete the study in a time- and resource-efficient manner (that is, to recruit enough individuals or the right types of individuals)? If there is no core questions that all sites will address, there is little reason to consider an MSE.

Interventions. Will the same interventions be employed at all sites? If not, one is clearly not going to be conducting a multicenter clinical trial. However, a number of other factors need to be considered before deciding on the appropriateness of conducting a different type of multiple site study. For example, when interventions vary markedly, pooling data may be inappropriate, and it may be more cost-efficient to conduct a number of individual studies that will then be synthesized using meta-analytic techniques. However, when one is interested in exploring the relative effectiveness of alternative interventions for similar populations, a multiple site evaluation with common outcome measures across sites may enable the evaluator to select one or two interventions that have greater impacts than the others.

Study Populations. Will the same inclusion and exclusion criteria be used across sites? If not, what is the reason for allowing differences? What impact will the variation have on data analyses? Any differences among sites in inclusion and exclusion criteria will lessen the comparability of study populations across sites. Furthermore, even if inclusion and exclusion criteria are similar across sites, population demography (such as age and gender distributions) and clinical characteristics (such as severity of illness) may still differ across sites. Variation can increase generalizability and external validity but can complicate data analysis and interpretations.

Evaluation Design. What requirements will be placed on sites in terms of evaluation design parameters (such as random assignment to conditions, type of control or comparison group, number and timing of assessments, instrumentation, or synchronization of implementation with other sites)? Within a clinical trials context, all of these elements are constrained by a standard protocol. With other MSEs, these design decisions may not be constrained. Variations in each of these areas inevitably lead to complications in data analysis and interpretation. A well-designed and well-implemented MSE should not only detect the impact of the intervention but will also allow for an exploration of the mediators and moderators of the impact. When clinical trial models are not employed, statistical techniques and the use of logic models can improve understanding of causal mechanisms (Davidson, 2000).

Coordination. How will the activities undertaken at the various sites be coordinated? The need to coordinate activities across the sites with MSEs (relative to studies in a single site) adds staffing, time, and financial costs to a study. Unless there are sufficient resources that can be devoted to the coordination of activities, one may want to question the appropriateness of conducting an MSE.

Training and Quality Assurance. How will adherence to the protocol across sites be ensured? This includes training (and retraining) for interviewers and treatment providers, assessing fidelity of the intervention, and monitoring data quality. Although costs for these activities are involved in any study, the costs for coordinating these activities across sites will add to the resources required.

Data Analysis. What strategy will be used to combine and centrally analyze the data collected across the various sites? It is important to note that the assumption in many multicenter clinical trials that the standardization across centers obviates any need to include differences across centers in the analysis of the data is now being increasingly questioned. A variety of data-analytic strategies exist to deal with potential between-site differences. A common approach to examining site issues within MSEs is to use hierarchical linear modeling to control for the random effect of programs beyond the fixed effects of client characteristics (Grella, Joshi, and Hser, 2000). This approach is particularly useful in MSEs in which both client characteristics and specific treatment approaches vary across sites. Choosing not to examine effects associated with sites seems unwise; unanalyzed site effects can obscure or exaggerate pooled findings, and ignoring contextual factors is a squandered opportunity.

Purpose of This Volume

The principal purpose of this volume is to explore the use of MSEs for evaluating the efficacy or effectiveness of interventions and to derive lessons to guide the planning and implementation of similar studies. We draw on the experiences of five MSEs funded by SAMHSA but seek to develop lessons for the field in general. The MSE examples described in this volume share a number of characteristics. First, each was funded for the explicit purpose of developing generalizable knowledge about the effectiveness of a defined intervention. Second, each involves the evaluation of one or more existing interventions or interventions implemented in association with the evaluation activity. Third, each involves two or more distinct geographical sites. Finally, each involves quantitative or qualitative comparisons made across sites by a third party. The MSE examples also differ in a number of important ways: in the number of sites, the number of interventions being tested, the source of the intervention being tested (research versus existing program), the organization of the program, the evaluation requirements placed on the sites, and many other factors. Chapter Seven, which draws on the experiences of the five multiple site evaluations, the available literature, and the experiences of the authors in other multiple site evaluations, synthesizes answers to the questions posed here and develops guidelines for the development and conduct of multiple site evaluations.

References

Barley, Z. A., and Jenness, M. "Cluster Evaluation: A Method to Strengthen Evaluation in Smaller Programs with Similar Purposes." *Evaluation Practice,* 1993, *14,* 141–147.

Davidson, E. J. "Ascertaining Causality in Theory-Based Evaluation." In P. J. Rogers, T. A. Hacsi, A. Petrosino, and T. A. Huebner (Eds.), *Program Theory in Evaluation: Challenges and Opportunities.* New Directions for Evaluation, no. 87. San Francisco: Jossey-Bass, 2000.

Dennis, M. L., Perl, H. I., Huebner, R. B., and McLellan, A. T. "Twenty-Five Strategies for Improving the Design, Implementation and Analysis of Health Services Research Related to Alcohol and Other Drug Abuse Treatment." *Addiction,* 2000, *95* (Suppl. 3), S281–S308.

Flay, B. R. "Efficacy and Effectiveness Trials (and Other Phases of Research) in the Development of Health Promotion Programs." *Preventive Medicine,* 1986, *15,* 451–474.

Friedman, L. M., Furberg, C. D., and DeMets, D. L. *Fundamentals of Clinical Trials.* (3rd ed.) New York: Springer-Verlag, 1998.

Grella, C. E., Joshi, V., and Hser, Y. "Program Variation in Treatment Outcomes Among Women in Residential Drug Treatment." *Evaluation Review,* 2000, *24,* 364–383.

Hanrahan, P., and others. "Cooperative Agreements for CMHS/CSAT Collaborative Program to Prevent Homelessness: Conclusion." *Alcoholism Treatment Quarterly,* 1999, *17,* 183–203.

Holder, H., and others. "Phases of Alcohol Problem Prevention Research." *Alcoholism: Clinical and Experimental Research,* 1999, *23,* 183–194.

Jainchill, N., Hawke, J., De Leon, G., and Yagelka, J. "Adolescents in Therapeutic Communities: One-Year Posttreatment Outcomes." *Journal of Psychoactive Drugs,* 2000, *32,* 81–94.

Kershaw, D., and Fair, J. *The New Jersey Income Maintenance Experiment.* Orlando, Fla.: Academic Press, 1976.

Kraemer, H. C. "Pitfalls of Multisite Randomized Clinical Trials of Efficacy and Effectiveness." *Schizophrenia Bulletin,* 2000, *26,* 533–541.

Meinert, C. L. *Clinical Trials: Design, Conduct, and Analysis.* New York: Oxford University Press, 1986.

Newhouse, J. P., and others. "Some Interim Results from a Controlled Trial of Cost Sharing in Health Insurance." *New England Journal of Medicine,* 1981, *305,* 1501–1507.

Sinacore, J. M., and Turpin, R. S. "Multiple Sites in Evaluation Research: A Survey of Organizational and Methodological Issues." In R. S. Turpin and J. M. Sinacore (Eds.), *Multisite Evaluations.* New Directions for Evaluation, no. 50. New York: Jossey-Bass, 1991.

Springer, F. "Lessons Learned from Multiple Cross-Site Evaluation Studies." Paper presented at the American Evaluation Association Meeting, Honolulu, Nov. 2000.

Straw, R. B., Levine, I. S., and Osher, F. C. "The Federal Role in Developing Solutions for Societal Problems." In W. R. Breakey and J. W. Thompson (Eds.), *Mentally Ill and Homeless: Special Programs for Special Needs.* Amsterdam: Harwood, 1997.

Tinsman, P. D., and others. "Factors Affecting Client Response to HIV Outreach Efforts." *Journal of Substance Abuse,* 2001, *13,* 201–214.

Turpin, R. S., and Sinacore, J. M. (Eds.). *Multisite Evaluations.* New Directions for Evaluation, no. 50. San Francisco: Jossey-Bass, 1991.

Williams, R. J., Chang, S. Y., and Addiction Centre Adolescent Research Group. "A Comprehensive and Comparative Review of Adolescent Substance Abuse Treatment Outcome." *Clinical Psychology: Science and Practice,* 2000, *7,* 138–166.

Worthen, B. R., and Schmitz, C. C. "Conceptual Challenges Confronting Cluster Evaluation." *Evaluation,* 1997, *3,* 300–310.

ROGER B. STRAW *is director of the Division of Planning and Evaluation, Office of Planning and Evaluation, Health Resources and Services Administration, U.S. Department of Health and Human Services.*

JAMES M. HERRELL *is a social science analyst with the Center for Substance Abuse Treatment, Substance Abuse and Mental Health Services Administration, U.S. Department of Health and Human Services.*

2

This chapter describes methodological and logistical issues associated with the design, development, and management of the Marijuana Treatment Project, a multisite, randomized clinical trial investigating the effectiveness of brief interventions for individuals who are dependent on marijuana.

Treating Marijuana Dependence in Adults: A Multisite, Randomized Clinical Trial

Thomas F. Babor, Karen L. Steinberg, Bonnie McRee, Janice Vendetti, Kathleen M. Carroll

Some multisite evaluations examine interventions that are implemented in the same way across all sites, whereas others evaluate different interventions across sites (Sinacore and Turpin, 1991). The study reported here, the Marijuana Treatment Project (MTP), a multisite evaluation initiated in 1996 by the Center for Substance Abuse Treatment (CSAT) within the Substance Abuse and Mental Health Services Administration, is an example of the former; it has the advantage of providing generalizable knowledge about the extent to which brief therapies for persons with marijuana dependence have similar effects on different subpopulations. MTP was conducted as a multisite clinical trial, a collaborative approach to clinical research that has become increasingly popular in the evaluation of many different kinds of medical and psychiatric treatments (Friedman, Furberg, and De Mets, 1998; Meinert, 1986). Because of their cost and complexity, relatively few multicenter clinical trials have been conducted to evaluate treatments for substance use disorders. Perhaps the most ambitious example of a multisite clinical trial of this type is Project MATCH, which evaluated treatment

This research was supported by grant no. 280–94–0008 from the Center for Substance Abuse Treatment and the Center for Mental Health Services, Substance Abuse and Mental Health Services Administration (SAMHSA), U.S. Department of Health and Human Services. The interpretations and conclusions presented in this chapter are the views of the authors and do not necessarily represent the official policy or position of SAMHSA.

matching with 1,726 alcoholics at ten sites (Babor and Del Boca, forthcoming). That trial encountered major challenges in terms of research design, assessment procedures, standardization of treatment, project management, and statistical analysis (Fuller and others, 1994; Carroll and others, 1994; McRee, 1998). In many respects, the experience gained from Project MATCH in the evaluation of manual-guided psychotherapy (that is, therapist services provided in accordance with a well-defined written protocol) provided a model for MTP. In this chapter, we describe the context of MTP from a knowledge development perspective, the rationale for the study's research design, the major challenges encountered in project implementation, and the lessons learned from conducting the trial.

Phase of Research

Multisite evaluations differ in important ways according to the phase of research they represent, ranging from descriptive and exploratory studies, designed to provide a preliminary understanding of a problem, to confirmatory and replication studies. Confirmatory studies involve the rigorous evaluation of a standardized effectiveness model, whereas replication studies examine the effectiveness of well-tested interventions under conditions of general use with different subpopulations or with different adaptations of the intervention. MTP represents both the confirmatory and replication phases of research. To the extent that prior research had established that behavioral therapies were effective for adults with marijuana dependence, the trial sought to confirm and extend these findings with different subpopulations and a more refined specification of the psychotherapy process.

In the mid-1990s, when MTP was conceived as a cooperative agreement under CSAT's Knowledge Development and Application program, national survey data were showing increasing prevalence of regular marijuana use in the United States. The National Co-Morbidity Study (Anthony, Warner, and Kessler, 1994) found that 4.2 percent of adults met lifetime criteria for cannabis dependence, and 1 percent of the population reported dependence symptoms in the past month. Although marijuana was once thought to be secondary to the abuse of other drugs or alcohol, clinical studies were identifying a group of primary marijuana users (Roffman, Stephens, Simpson, and Whitaker, 1988; Stephens, Roffman, and Simpson, 1993), who present for treatment with marijuana as their main and often only drug of abuse.

Despite the high prevalence of regular marijuana use and dependence, as well as the growing evidence of harmful effects (Hall and Babor, 2000), there has been relatively little research on how best to treat persons with marijuana dependence. Most researchers have adapted other drug treatment or general psychotherapy approaches to the marijuana-abusing population. Cognitive-behavioral approaches have been commonly used (Stephens,

Roffman, and Simpson, 1994). The cognitive-behavioral perspective views substance abuse as a maladaptive way of coping with problems or meeting certain needs. As with any other learned behavior pattern, cannabis abuse should be susceptible to alteration through the application of behavior modification interventions.

Other approaches have focused on social support as a key in helping people to overcome drug dependence (Stephens, Roffman, and Simpson, 1994). Length of time or intensity of treatment has not been addressed in the literature. There has been little systematic study of treatment process parameters, such as therapist characteristics and the client-therapist relationship, especially with specific reference to treating marijuana dependence.

Because of the lack of research on treatment for cannabis dependence and the potential benefits of studying both brief and extended cognitive-behavioral relapse-prevention therapies, MTP was designed to generate new information about the effectiveness of focused treatment for marijuana dependence and to replicate the results of previous single-site studies. It was reasoned that if the results were positive, the manual-guided therapies developed for this project should be readily transferable to specialized outpatient clinics and primary care practitioners.

Project Description

Under the terms of this cooperative agreement, researchers defined the details of the project within the guidelines of the Guidance for Applicants announcing the grant program, agreeing to accept close coordination and guidance by the project's steering committee in all aspects of scientific and technical management. CSAT staff collaborated with the investigators and had substantial programmatic involvement. MTP was a three-year, randomized clinical trial to investigate the effectiveness of brief interventions for individuals who are dependent on marijuana. Working with CSAT program staff and consultants, the coordinating center and site investigators formed a steering committee to develop a workable research design, construct detailed treatment manuals, choose appropriate assessment instruments, and conduct a pilot study before implementing the trial. The study sought to answer two primary questions: (1) Are brief interventions more effective than no treatment for marijuana problems (referral to a waiting list control)? (2) Does a nine-session episode of treatment produce outcomes superior to a two-session treatment? Experienced and specially trained therapists delivered the treatments. Four hundred fifty chronic marijuana smokers representing diverse socioeconomic and ethnic backgrounds were recruited through media advertisements and agency referrals.

Study Design. MTP investigated the efficacy of two short-term interventions in varying populations of individuals who were dependent on cannabis. The three collaborating sites collectively recruited 450 participants (308 men and 142 women). The sample reported an average of 18.0 years of regular marijuana use (defined as three or more times a week) and 9.2 years of problem use, which was measured by asking respondents to estimate the age at which they first experienced the kinds of problems that led them to seek treatment.

The study sample at each site was randomly assigned to three study protocols using individual (rather than group) therapy on an outpatient basis: a two-session brief intervention, a nine-session extended treatment, or a delayed-treatment control group.

The rationale for a multisite trial of outpatient treatments was based on practical and theoretical considerations. On a practical level, the three institutions funded to participate in the trial provide access to different types of participants with varying socioeconomic backgrounds. Because much of the published research on therapies for cannabis dependence was carried out primarily with male, Caucasian, employed individuals, special attention was devoted to the recruitment of women, ethnic minorities, and persons who were unemployed.

The selection of two brief treatment conditions was based on the desirability of combining a range of promising or currently available treatment approaches (motivational enhancement therapy, coping skills training based on a relapse-prevention model, and case management approaches). Individual treatments were used because it is difficult to study therapeutic processes in group therapy and because group therapy is not recommended for small numbers of sessions.

Participants assigned to the two-session intervention received treatment over a five-week period, and those randomized to the more intensive nine-session therapy were seen over a twelve-week period. Participants assigned to the two treatment conditions were evaluated at four, nine, and fifteen months after the start of treatment. In addition, follow-up interviews were conducted by telephone twenty-one months after the start of treatment. The primary assessment for the delayed-treatment control group was conducted at the four-month follow-up point (after randomization). This follow-up allowed for assessment of the delayed-treatment control group condition after participants in both active treatments had gone at least one month without treatment. The primary outcome measure was the frequency of marijuana use during the assessment period.

Participants in the active treatment conditions were also assessed at the end of treatment, which occurred approximately five weeks and three months after the start of treatment for the brief and extended treatment conditions, respectively. These brief assessments collected only essential information at the end of treatment (for example, global assessment of marijuana use during the last weeks of treatment and evaluations of treatment) and were conducted by telephone for persons who did not attend the last treatment session. The delayed-treatment control group was assessed at four and twelve weeks after randomization to maintain contact with participants and to identify signs of clinical deterioration.

Main Findings. Findings obtained from follow-up evaluations at four months after the initiation of treatment indicated significant improvements in both treatment groups relative to the control group, with the nine-session group showing better outcomes than the two-session group at all subsequent follow-up evaluations conducted at nine, fifteen, and twenty-one months (MTP Research Group, 2002). These results, based on self-report data, were replicated with urine toxicology data. These significant treatment effects were also seen for secondary outcome measures, including depression, marijuana-related problems, and dependence symptoms. No differential effects of treatment by gender, ethnicity, or employment status were found, suggesting that the interventions were equally effective with special population groups. Further analyses using the nine- and fifteen-month follow-up data indicated that the nine-session treatment reduced marijuana smoking significantly, with little deterioration of the treatment effects over time. No significant site-by-treatment condition interactions were observed.

Issues and Resolutions

Several features of the trial presented organizational, ethical, and methodological challenges to the study team. The first two issues summarized in Table 2.1 are specific to multisite evaluations, whereas the others are more generic to randomized clinical trials, whether conducted at one site or many sites. First, the cooperative agreement was funded for a three-year period. This relatively short funding period placed significant constraints on the planning and initiation of the study, the duration of participant recruitment, and the length of the follow-up evaluation. Second, the standardization of diagnostic assessments and therapy implementation across sites required special attention. If the clinical data were not collected consistently across sites, systematic bias could have been introduced, resulting in site differences in outcomes. Similarly, the training and supervision of therapists were

Table 2.1. Issues and Resolutions in the Marijuana Treatment Project

Issues	Nature of Issue	Resolutions
Rapid implementation	Organizational	Steering committee
Cross-site standardization	Methodological, organizational	Research assistants and therapist training and supervision
Control group	Methodological, ethical	Delayed treatment, control group
Balanced comparison groups	Methodological	Urn randomization conducted centrally by coordinating center
Adequate follow-up rate	Methodological	Compliance enhancement procedures
Clinical deterioration	Ethical	Monitoring protocol
Valid and reliable measurements	Methodological	Use of standardized tests and validity enhancement techniques

major issues in the implementation of the trial, requiring special efforts in the design of the treatment protocols and the oversight provided during the delivery of interventions. Third, the need for an untreated control group, balanced comparison groups, a sufficient follow-up rate, and a protocol for monitoring clinical deterioration created logistical, ethical, and methodological challenges. Another difficulty was the selection of reliable and valid measurement instruments, especially those capable of providing corroboration of information collected with self-report methods. Because of the skepticism expressed by critics of self-report methods, it was necessary to use alternative measurement techniques that provided a check on the participants' verbal report of marijuana use.

Rapid Implementation. To address the implementation challenges, the steering committee adopted a participatory process of collaborative problem solving. During the initial planning phase, MTP established an organizational structure that allowed the three clinical research units (CRUs), the coordinating center, and CSAT to function collaboratively. This group was responsible for the overall direction of the study, development of the trial protocol, implementation of the protocol at each CRU, monitoring study progress, development of collaboration policies (for example, publications and data access), and reporting of study results. All major decisions were determined by a majority vote of the steering committee. The CSAT project officer was responsible for monitoring the conduct of the study and for fiscal management of the project. Two working groups were formed: one to develop and monitor the treatment interventions and another to plan and execute the research design. The groups worked quickly to achieve consensus, building on the experience of the project's consultants and investigators. Therapist manuals were written and pilot-tested, and standardized assessment instruments were selected. A major challenge was the need to recruit sufficient numbers of participants to provide enough statistical power to test the study hypotheses, taking into account site effects and subgroup differences. A variety of effective techniques were used to recruit participants and monitor their progress up to twenty-one months after the initiation of treatment. Because much of the research on therapies for marijuana dependence was conducted with male, Caucasian, employed samples, the current study was interested in populations with higher proportions of ethnic minorities, unemployed persons, and women. Specific outreach strategies were used to recruit a higher proportion of minority participants. These included gender- and minority-specific advertising campaigns, employment of female and minority therapists and research staff, and outreach efforts using local media and public service announcements.

To monitor study progress across sites located in different parts of the country, the coordinating center developed mechanisms to provide CRUs and CSAT with timely information about the characteristics of the sample and the progress of the trial. Such reports were essential for identifying problems as they arose. In addition to sending data files to the coordinating center on a monthly basis, each CRU had to provide monthly reports that included (1) statistics on participant recruitment (for example, number of persons screened, number of participants enrolled in the trial, reasons for exclusion), (2) data on participant retention, and (3) participant compliance (for example, number of therapy sessions attended, number of baseline evaluations completed, number of follow-up assessments completed).

The monthly CRU reports and the data files were used to generate quarterly reports that contained both individual site and trial-wide statistics. The report was designed not only to describe the study's progress, but to motivate sites to achieve the trial's recruitment goals, identify problems encountered in protocol implementation, and suggest possible changes in policies and procedures.

Cross-Site Standardization. The standardization of data collection and intervention procedures is a major challenge in multisite evaluations. Inconsistent application of study procedures, such as interviewing techniques or follow-up protocols, could compromise the internal validity of the study. Similarly, the specificity and effectiveness of the study intervention could be affected by differences across sites in the therapists' behavior. For these reasons, special attention was devoted in MTP to the training of research staff and therapists.

Research assistants were trained and routinely monitored by the coordinating center. Training focused on the correct procedures for screening potential participants, conducting structured diagnostic interviews, administering tests and questionnaires, conducting follow-up interviews, and cleaning and entering data. At the onset of the trial, a three-day seminar was conducted to train project coordinators and research staff. Project coordinators at each site then trained newly hired research assistants at CRUs. Reliability checking and supervision were conducted both on- and off-site throughout the study. So that interviewer ratings remained reliable over time, periodic checks were made of each interviewer at each site using audiotaped recordings.

Control Group. The delayed-treatment control condition was a scientific requirement that presented logistical and ethical challenges. Without a control group, causal inferences could not be made about the number and nature of the changes in marijuana use resulting from the treatment interventions.

A waiting list control group has several advantages. It permits the eventual delivery of a therapeutic intervention to participants who are in need of treatment, while at the same time providing a basis for comparing the active interventions. If designed correctly, the waiting list control group can provide valuable information about the amount of change in marijuana use and its consequences that could be expected in the normal course of time, independent of a specific treatment intervention. However, two problems that complicated the use of a waiting list control group were the possibility of differential attrition in the control group and the ethical dilemma of withholding treatment for a relatively long period of time, during which treatments were delivered and evaluated with other participants.

To address these problems, we limited the duration of the waiting period to four months. Delayed-treatment control participants were scheduled to receive the treatment of their choice following the four-month follow-up assessment. During the recruitment phase, all participants were screened to determine their capacity to delay receiving treatment without ill effects. No research volunteers were deemed ineligible by the CRU project coordinators because they required immediate treatment. Research staff contacted each participant assigned to the waiting list condition four and twelve weeks after randomization. These contacts served the dual purposes of updating locator information collected at the initial assessment and evaluating participants for deterioration in their drug use, mental status, and physical health that would indicate the need for immediate intervention. Any participant who asked questions or expressed concerns about continuing to wait for treatment was put in contact with the designated clinical staff member, who assessed the need for referral to immediate treatment. It should be noted that marijuana use, even at levels leading to dependence, has not been shown to be life threatening. In the light of the eighteen years of regular marijuana use reported by the research participants, the four-month delay of treatment was not likely to add significantly to the risk of disease or other consequences.

Balanced Comparison Groups. A major challenge in all clinical trials is the creation of balanced comparison groups that are similar in terms of prognostic factors likely to influence the study outcomes. Although random assignment is the typical procedure for creating similar groups across experimental conditions, it is not unusual for groups to differ on several potential confounding factors after randomization. To address this problem, the study used an urn randomization procedure to maximize the probability that the treatment groups were comparable with regard to characteristics deemed likely to affect the outcome of the study (Stout, Wirtz, Carbonari, and Del Boca, 1994). In this probabilistic balancing procedure, the balancing variables were severity of marijuana problems, age, gender, employment status, ethnicity, and education.

The process of randomization was conducted centrally at the coordinating center with a computer program to prevent the introduction of any assignment bias at the local sites. Intakes at each recruitment site were balanced separately so that each CRU constituted a balanced substudy. CRUs notified the coordinating center when they had a candidate for randomization. Each CRU provided identifying information (not including name), values for all the balancing factors, and certification that the participant met eligibility criteria. Within one business day, the coordinating center reported back to each CRU the participant's treatment assignment.

Follow-Up Rate. Randomized trials in substance abuse research strive for an adequate follow-up rate to improve generalizability of findings and to avoid the biasing effect of differential attrition across groups. A rate of 70 percent is considered minimal, 80 percent is adequate, and 90 percent is good (Fuller and others, 1994). Several procedures were used to ensure adequate follow-up rates at the successive follow-up points (Zweben and others, 1998): informing the participant of the importance of follow-up evaluations at the time of the initial assessment; describing the role expectations of a research participant; guaranteeing complete confidentiality of all information; obtaining addresses, telephone numbers, and other information needed for tracking participants; arranging for home visits and telephone interviews when participants failed to keep appointments; developing rapport between participants and research assistants; mailing of appointment reminders that were followed by telephone calls; and provision of incentive payments for the successful completion of follow-up evaluations.

So that compliance improved with follow-up, participants in the treatment conditions were paid fifty dollars for each of their primary follow-up appointments (at four and nine months). The delayed-treatment control participants were paid fifty dollars for their four-month follow-up interview. These payments were intended to defray the costs of transportation to the interview site and to compensate participants for their time and inconvenience.

Clinical Deterioration. Clinical researchers have an ethical responsibility to ensure that their treatments do no harm and that research participants receive optimal care during their participation in the study. Procedures were developed for the CRU staff to withdraw a participant from the treatment protocol in case of significant deterioration in clinical condition. The criteria developed to guide this decision applied to the participant's condition during both active treatment and the waiting list control period. It was difficult to define deterioration in terms of marijuana use alone. Participants may experience deterioration along a number of different (although potentially interrelated) dimensions that could contribute to their being removed from the active treatment protocol (but not from the outcome follow-up assessments): acute psychosis; suicidal or homicidal ideation, intent, or plan; violent behavior; onset of significant cognitive impairment or disorientation; serious deterioration of physical health; arrest and incarceration that would prevent continuation in treatment; and alcohol or drug use resulting in adverse consequences and the need for inpatient hospitalization. Fortunately, no participants were withdrawn from participation because of clinical deterioration.

Validity of Self-Reports. Many validity enhancement procedures were used to improve the accuracy of self-report data (Babor, Brown, and Del Boca, 1990): clear instructions to participants emphasizing the need for accurate data; the use of standardized, well-validated assessment instruments; differentiating the participants' role as research subjects from their role as patients; and the use of urine screen tests as a "bogus pipeline" to suggest the possibility of independent verification of verbal report data. In addition, we were able to achieve independent verification of some key outcome measures by means of collateral reports and urine toxicology testing.

Collateral verification of marijuana use was obtained for a random sample of approximately one-third (36 percent) of the participants who completed the follow-up assessments. Collateral verification came from spouses or partners (56 percent), other relatives (15 percent), or friends (29 percent) of the participants. One hundred percent of those who reported complete abstinence during the four-month follow-up were verified by their collateral informant, whereas 91 percent who reported smoking marijuana during this time period were in agreement with their informant. The 9 percent in disagreement occurred because the collateral informant reported abstinence when the participant reported smoking.

To provide additional validation of self-report data, we obtained urine specimens for all participants at each of the primary data collection points (baseline and four- and nine-month assessments). Enzyme immunoassay tests were used as a screen, and quantitative analyses were conducted on all positive screenings with gas chromatography–mass spectrometry. The qualitative screening results were compared with self-reported marijuana use during the two-week period before the specimen was collected. Percentage agreement was very high for each time point (94 percent at baseline, 91 percent at four months, 92 percent at nine months). As with the collateral data, most discrepancies occurred because participants reported marijuana use when the urine screening indicated that the participant was abstinent. The urine specimen results and collateral informant data both suggest that participants did not systematically underreport their use of marijuana.

Therapist Training, Supervision, and Monitoring. Therapist training, supervision, and monitoring involved initial screening of applicants for the therapist positions, centralized training of the therapists, and monitoring therapists' behavior over the course of the study to ensure adherence and competence with regard to the study treatments. Therapists from the different sites were brought together for a three-day training seminar at the coordinating center. The curriculum for this seminar covered two major areas: explication, demonstration, and role playing of therapeutic methods outlined in the training manuals and procedures for conducting psychotherapy within the context of a clinical trial.

Centralized training and monitoring were designed to maximize the precision of the treatments being offered and minimize the degree to which cross-site differences occurred. A critical part of the standardization process was the use of detailed therapist manuals describing each type of treatment, including underlying theoretical bases, recommended sequencing of therapeutic tasks, session content, and practical examples of implementation.

To minimize the possibility that study treatments might be adversely affected by unskilled or inexperienced therapists, we hired only experienced therapists. To allow consistent cross-site implementation of each type of psychotherapy, centralized training staff conducted continuing supervision. All sessions were videotaped, and randomly selected tapes were sent to the training site. The supervisor at the training site rated the entire session before the next supervisory session. Supervision took place on a regular basis, consisting of sixty-minute telephone calls in which supervisor rating forms were reviewed. These forms were composed of items assessing treatment fidelity, as well as therapist competence with specific therapeutic tasks and general, nonspecific therapy skills (for example, empathy, concern, therapeutic relationship). In addition to telephone supervision with the training site supervisors, therapists at each site met monthly as a group. During the training phase, the supervisor reviewed videotapes of every session and provided one hour of supervision per week for every study therapist. After the training phase, contact between the coordinating center and treatment sites continued on a less intensive schedule. If these monitoring procedures detected instances where the therapist was deviating significantly from the study treatments as described in the training manuals, supervisors had the option to schedule additional supervision sessions.

A centralized process study was conducted to evaluate the degree to which the different treatments were delivered consistently and to monitor adherence to the principles underlying each of the treatments. Most of the process ratings were made by session tape observers, who were blind to the participant's study condition. In addition, the quality of the therapeutic alliance was rated from multiple perspectives (observer, participant, and therapist). A review of 633 sessions, representing 164 participants, by independent evaluators blind to the subjects' treatment condition indicated that therapists closely adhered to the standardized manuals throughout treatment. There were no significant differences across the three sites in treatment adherence or competence or in other process indicators, such as the working alliance (Carroll and others, 2002).

Lessons Learned

The lessons learned from the design and execution of MTP include the value of collaborative decision making, the need for scientific rigor in the research design and data collection, the benefits of using manual-guided therapies, the importance of follow-up compliance techniques, and the advantages of multisite evaluation studies.

The first lesson pertains to management style. The participatory and collaborative process of decision making helped to minimize the conflict that sometimes develops between an autocratic coordinating center and passive clinical sites. By involving site personnel in planning and decision making, the MTP coordinating center was able to accomplish a large number of complex tasks within a tight time frame. Although investigators on many occasions held differing viewpoints about important aspects of the trial (for example, how to implement a control group, how to handle randomization with pregnant participants), the early meetings and frequent conference calls fostered relationship building among members of the steering committee and provided a forum to resolve differences and maintain a common vision.

The traditional model of the multicenter randomized clinical trial is considered the gold standard for scientific evaluation of therapeutic interventions (Meinert, 1986). Nevertheless, it can be subject to the same threats to internal validity as quasi-experimental studies, especially when conducted in the form of multisite evaluations. MTP incorporated a number of methodological safeguards designed to increase the validity of the study: a waiting list control group, cross-site standardization measures, urn randomization to balance comparison groups, the use of standardized assessments, and validity enhancement procedures. These safeguards seemed to increase the quality of the data collected and the confidence that could be placed in the findings. The lack of site differences on any of the study's outcome measures is an indication of the benefit of these procedures.

There is a general assumption that randomized clinical trials are more relevant to efficacy questions (for example, is there a causal relationship between the intervention and the outcome?) than effectiveness questions (for example, does the relationship replicate under real-world conditions?) because of their emphasis on internal versus external validity. Although there is truth to this assumption, we found in MTP that it is quite possible to conduct a multisite evaluation with a heterogeneous sample in community treatment settings. Moreover, it is possible not only to generalize to diverse populations, but to address effectiveness questions as well. Our experience with conducting the trial and developing a systematic training manual for our research therapists translated directly to the publication of a treatment manual (Steinberg and others, forthcoming) and a related training package, which permit rapid dissemination of the new treatment technologies to practitioners in the field.

Another important lesson from this trial, which relates directly to issues of effectiveness and generalizability of findings, involves the use of a manual-guided, as opposed to manual-driven, approach to the delivery of study treatments. Investigators encouraged therapists to integrate the theoretical framework of the study therapies into their work with participants, but they were told not to deliver therapy in a prescribed way, as though following a recipe for therapeutic intervention. It can be a difficult balance to achieve, but we found that therapists were able to deliver core therapeutic components without compromising their own style of conducting psychotherapy. We thought that this would increase the degree to which the treatments could be readily translated into community settings.

Conclusion

MTP indicates that carefully controlled multisite evaluations need not be so artificial that their results are irrelevant to routine clinical practice. Our experience with MTP indicates that multisite evaluations have definite advantages over smaller, single-site clinical trials because they make possible the rapid recruitment of a large and diverse sample. Collaboration among a group of investigators permits the division of labor and expertise to maximize design quality and creative decision making. Finally, the combination of methodological rigor and clinical relevance in a rapidly executed multisite evaluation has the added advantage of translating scientific findings into treatment policy because the results are often timely and unambiguous.

References

Anthony, J. C., Warner, L. A., and Kessler, R. C. "Comparative Epidemiology of Dependence on Tobacco, Alcohol, Controlled Substances, and Inhalants: Basic Findings from the National Comorbidity Survey." *Experimental and Clinical Psychopharmacology*, 1994, 2, 244–268.

Babor, T., Brown, J., and Del Boca, F. "Validity of Self-Reports in Applied Research on Addictive Behaviors: Fact or Fiction?" *Behavioral Assessment*, 1990, 12, 5–31.

Babor, T., and Del Boca, F. K. (Eds.). *Treatment Matching in Alcoholism*. Cambridge: Cambridge University Press, forthcoming.

Carroll, K. M., and others. "Implementing Treatment and Protecting the Validity of the Independent Variable in Treatment Matching Studies." *Journal of Studies on Alcohol*, 1994, 12 (Suppl.), 149–155.

Carroll, K. M., and others. "Process and Outcome in a Multisite Trial of Treatments for Marijuana Dependence." Unpublished manuscript, 2002.

Friedman, L. M., Furberg, C. D., and DeMets, D. L. *Fundamentals of Clinical Trials*. (3rd ed.). New York: Springer-Verlag, 1998.

Fuller, R. K., and others. "Multisite Clinical Trials in Alcoholism Treatment Research: Organizational, Methodological and Management Issues." *Journal of Studies on Alcohol*, 1994, 12, 30–37.

Hall, W., and Babor, T. F. "Cannabis Use and Public Health: Assessing the Burden." *Addiction*, 2000, 95, 485–490.

Marijuana Treatment Project Research Group. "Treating Cannabis Dependence: Findings from a Randomized Trial." Unpublished manuscript, 2002.

McRee, B. "The Role of a Coordinating Center in Facilitating Research Compliance in a Multisite Clinical Trial." In A. Zweben and others (Eds.), *Strategies for Facilitating Protocol Compliance in Alcoholism Treatment Research*. Bethesda, Md.: National Institute on Alcohol Abuse and Alcoholism, 1998.

Meinert, C. L. *Clinical Trials: Design, Conduct, and Analysis*. New York: Oxford University Press, 1986.

Roffman, R. A., Stephens, R. S., Simpson, E. E., and Whitaker, D. L. "Treatment of Marijuana Dependence: Preliminary Results." *Journal of Psychoactive Drugs*, 1988, 20, 129–137.

Sinacore, J. M., and Turpin, R. S. "Multiple Sites in Evaluation Research: A Survey of Organizational and Methodological Issues." In R. S. Turpin and J. M. Sinacore (Eds.), *Multisite Evaluations*. New Directions for Evaluation, no. 50. San Francisco: Jossey-Bass, 1991.

Steinberg, K., and others (Eds.). *Brief Marijuana Dependence Counseling*. Rockville, Md.: Center for Substance Abuse Treatment, forthcoming.

Stephens, R. S., Roffman, R. A., and Simpson, E. E. "Adult Marijuana Users Seeking Treatment." *Journal of Consulting and Clinical Psychology*, 1993, 61, 1100–1104.

Stephens, R. S., Roffman, R. A., and Simpson, E. E. "Treating Adult Marijuana Dependence: A Test of the Relapse Prevention Model." *Journal of Consulting and Clinical Psychology*, 1994, 62, 92–99.

Stout, R. L., Wirtz, P. W., Carbonari, J. P., and Del Boca, F. K. "Ensuring Balanced Distribution of Prognostic Factors in Treatment Outcome Research." *Journal of Studies on Alcohol,* 1994, *12* (Suppl.), 70–75.

Zweben, A., and others. (Eds.). *Strategies for Facilitating Protocol Compliance in Alcoholism Treatment Research.* Bethesda, Md.: National Institute of Alcohol Abuse and Alcoholism, 1998.

THOMAS F. BABOR *is a professor and chair of the Department of Community Medicine and Health Care at the University of Connecticut School of Medicine, Farmington.*

KAREN L. STEINBERG *is an assistant professor in the Department of Psychiatry at the University of Connecticut School of Medicine, Farmington.*

BONNIE MCREE *is a research associate in the Department of Community Medicine and Health Care at the University of Connecticut School of Medicine, Farmington.*

JANICE VENDETTI *is a research associate in the Department of Community Medicine and Health Care at the University of Connecticut School of Medicine, Farmington.*

KATHLEEN M. CARROLL *is a professor in the Department of Psychiatry at Yale University School of Medicine, New Haven, Connecticut.*

3

The importance of close and effective collaboration to the success of a multisite study is the focus of this chapter, which describes the ways in which key parties worked together to identify and overcome the challenges of a large and complicated evaluation.

The Pioneer: The Employment Intervention Demonstration Program

Judith A. Cook, Martha Ann Carey, Lisa A. Razzano, Jane Burke, Crystal R. Blyler

The Employment Intervention Demonstration Program (EIDP) is a research demonstration program for the delivery and evaluation of innovative vocational interventions for mental health consumers. Funded in 1995 by the Center for Mental Health Services (CMHS) of the Substance Abuse and Mental Health Services Administration (SAMHSA), EIDP is administered through cooperative agreements with eight sites and a coordinating center. The program's purpose is to develop knowledge and policy-relevant information that address questions of national significance regarding the employment of individuals with severe mental illness. This encompasses the production of research findings that key mental health stakeholder groups (especially federal, state, and local policymakers and mental health consumers, providers, and advocates) can use to enhance the vocational potential of people with psychiatric disabilities. This chapter describes the development and progress of the program, a pioneering effort within SAMHSA and CMHS, and how its design and management enhanced the quality and policy relevance of the knowledge developed.

This research was funded by cooperative agreement SM51820 from the Center for Mental Health Services, Substance Abuse and Mental Health Services Administration. The views expressed are those of the authors and do not necessarily reflect the policy or position of any federal agency.

Genesis of the Employment Intervention Demonstration Program

In 1993, with input from mental health consumers, researchers, service providers, and families, CMHS identified the topic of employment as a focus for knowledge development. This choice stemmed from the importance of employment to persons with severe mental illness, many of whom live in poverty and identify work as an important life goal (Cook and Razzano, 2000), as well as the need for more empirical evidence regarding the relative effectiveness of different vocational rehabilitation models. Because the career patterns of persons with serious mental illness often are characterized by repeated cycles of employment followed by unemployment, a long-term perspective was deemed necessary, and the five-year initiative was designed to include a two-year follow-up period of data collection for all study participants.

At the time of EIDP's initial design, the state of the science in the psychiatric vocational rehabilitation field was such that numerous vocational rehabilitation models had been developed and tested through many valid and reliable measures. Some models had been evaluated with random assignment, and others had been studied with multivariate statistical approaches. However, little was known about the relative effectiveness of different models or about how well individual models worked in different environments and for different groups of service users. This state of knowledge justified the development of a multisite effectiveness study (Cook, 1995) in which models with demonstrated efficacy (that is, those evaluated under ideal conditions in laboratory-like settings) would be transferred to field-based settings and studied through random assignment to real-world service delivery programs operating in local communities.

Organized as a collaboration between federal personnel and researchers, EIDP was the first SAMHSA program designed to incorporate a multisite study within a series of site-specific, individual, stand-alone studies. The mechanism through which this occurred was the development of a common protocol of research instruments and procedures, which was created collaboratively by a multisite coordinating center, individual site representatives, federal government representatives, and consumers. Two other options were considered in developing the EIDP design: individual sites serving only as data collectors for a multisite study and a series of individual, unrelated studies, the approach previously used by the agency. The multisite plus stand-alone study design was selected to maximize what could be learned from individual studies as well as from combining data across studies, thus advancing scientific knowledge and realizing the knowledge development component of the overall Knowledge Development and Application (KDA) initiative of SAMHSA (see Chapter One, this volume).

EIDP was housed in the Community Support Program of CMHS, traditionally a source of support to states for the development and planning of public mental health systems. The KDA focus was new to the program and elicited a different type of application and different types of applicants. To have credible and useful service research results, the projects were required to use the most rigorous evaluation designs, such as random assignment, fidelity assessments of service interventions, establishment and maintenance of interrater reliability, and complex multivariate statistical analysis plans. The application component of the KDA process necessitated sophisticated dissemination plans targeted at a wide variety of stakeholder groups using a multitude of knowledge exchange modalities, particularly on the part of the coordinating center.

EIDP was funded in June 1995 with the selection of a coordinating center and four research projects, located in Maryland, Connecticut, South Carolina, and Pennsylvania. Because of the high quality of several unfunded applications, additional funds were allocated to add new projects (located in Arizona, Massachusetts, Maine, and Texas) in the third month of EIDP. The coordinating center is based at the Mental Health Services Research Program at the University of Illinois at Chicago, in partnership with the Human Services Research Institute located in Cambridge, Massachusetts. The funding announcement (Request for Applications SM 94–00) specified that the program's governance body would be a steering committee composed of the principal investigator from each project, the principal investigator of the coordinating center, consumers, and federal staff. Decisions were to be made collaboratively, through consensus if possible, and by a democratic vote (with one vote for each site, the federal staff, the coordinating center, state mental health representatives, and a consumer representative) when agreements were not unanimous.

Federal Role. Government personnel in a cooperative agreement have two distinct functions: (1) in the role of a federal program director, collaborating as a professional peer serving on a project steering committee, and (2) in the more traditional role of government project officer, monitoring the progress of individual projects and the overall program, as well as making recommendations for funding continuation. For EIDP, one person served in both roles. As a professional peer, the federal program director provided consultation and technical assistance to the overall program and to individual studies, including advice about instrument development and refinement, logic model development, analysis plans, fidelity measures, and recruitment and retention of research participants and staff. The management challenge for federal personnel involved guiding EIDP's progress in accord with CMHS's purpose, the needs and capabilities of the grantees, and the requirements of rigorous effectiveness research.

Role of Consumers. During the first year of the initiative, the steering committee voted to include a consumer-researcher as a voting member. Midway through the fourth year, in keeping with the increasing priority given by CMHS to involving consumers in all aspects of its work, this individual organized a consumer assembly, consisting of eight to fifteen consumers who had been involved in the study's management (that is, in roles other than research subject) at EIDP sites. With financial support from CMHS delivered through the coordinating center, the consumer assembly was convened by the steering committee consumer representative. With administrative support from the consumer-run Kentucky Center for Mental Health Studies, the assembly was convened through teleconferences and e-mail to solicit diverse consumers' opinions regarding EIDP; these opinions were then presented to the steering committee for consideration. Roles of the consumer assembly have included hypothesis development, examination and interpretation of preliminary findings, qualitative and case study analyses, identification of policy-related issues resulting from EIDP, and the development of products that might affect future employment studies and dissemination strategies. The later work of the group included building a national network to disseminate EIDP results to the community of consumer advocates, assisting in the refinement of definitions of outcomes, and developing questions regarding the processes of career development, such as impact of disclosure, or links between supported employment and educational programs.

Role of the Sites. Similar to more traditional single-site studies, each site was responsible for developing, implementing, and evaluating its chosen employment intervention. As a condition of funding, each site also agreed to cooperate with the development of the common protocol, in some cases reallocating staff and financial resources and modifying original study designs. The diverse experiences and perspectives of the different sites, along with their varying theoretical and methodological orientations, contributed to the multidisciplinary nature of EIDP and strengthened its overall quality. Individual sites contributed unique ideas that were incorporated into the overall study, such as conducting a rigorous assessment of study subjects' symptomatology, the need to monitor changes in quality of life co-occurring with employment, and the importance of assessing participant characteristics related to parenthood status and child care responsibilities. This made EIDP a whole that was more than the sum of its parts and proved to be a hallmark advantage to the collaborative multisite approach.

Role of the Coordinating Center. The multisite component of EIDP was designed so that a central role in its operation was played by the coordinating center, working in concert with the steering committee. The coordinating center was charged with overseeing the creation of the common protocol, consisting of a uniform set of research instruments, research procedures, interviewer training procedures, and data reporting strategies. This activity involved locating and distributing potential research instruments to sites for consideration, compiling and pilot-testing numerous drafts of the common protocol and documentation, coordinating initial and ongoing training in common data collection procedures, maintaining a record of group policy and procedure decisions, and operating an Internet listserv to facilitate steering committee communication and decision making.

Other responsibilities included the quarterly collection of common protocol data from all sites, ongoing monitoring of data quality, and analysis of longitudinal data on outcomes, services, satisfaction, and costs to address the major research questions of the multisite study.

Development of the Common Protocol

At its initial meetings, the steering committee reviewed each site's proposed vocational interventions, study designs, research instrumentation, sample sizes and power analyses, and assessment intervals and time frames. At subsequent meetings, the steering committee reached agreements about the cross-site study sample's inclusion and exclusion criteria, target populations, common study recruitment procedures, domains to be operationalized, instruments to measure each domain, length and order of the common protocol, and protocol administration.

Instrument Development. After an extensive review of instruments to measure work motivation among people with psychiatric disability, the steering committee decided that the lack of a valid, reliable measure of this important construct warranted the creation of a new instrument. Drawing from several previously published scales, coordinating center staff worked with the government program director and site principal investigators to adapt, pilot-test, and refine an instrument. Psychometric analyses of the scale data are now being readied for publication. To accurately assess negative symptoms that were hypothesized to be related to vocational outcomes, the steering committee voted to include in the common protocol the Positive and Negative Syndrome Scale (PANSS), requiring extensive training of EIDP interviewers (Kay, Opler, and Fishbein, 1986).

Working collaboratively with the steering committee, the coordinating center prepared and revised drafts of the Common Protocol Client Baseline and Six-Month Assessment and its accompanying documentation, the Employment Tracking Forms and the Clinician Rating Form, which is used to extract case record information and record assessments by clinicians. After the common protocol had been developed and pilot-tested, the coordinating center organized a three-day training session on general interviewing techniques, using the University of Michigan Survey Research Laboratory Interviewer Training procedures, manual, and tapes. Also included was training on administration of the PANSS and the Quality of Life Scale, delivered by the scales' authors and their associates. Concurrently, the Common Protocol computerized database structure was developed, tested, revised, and disseminated to project sites by coordinating center staff, along with a protocol for subject-client tracking.

Instrument Validation. Charged with responsibility for monitoring cross-site consistency and reliability, the coordinating center convened a psychometric panel of external consultants, who met with the steering committee to discuss validity and reliability analyses for the Common Protocol.

Working together, these groups developed a plan for collecting and analyzing test data from each of the eight sites to assess interrater reliability and the test-retest reliability of all previously published assessments that had been included in the Common Protocol. The psychometric panel then conducted analyses of the initial psychometric data, with positive results allowing data collection with the Common Protocol to proceed. The psychometric panel prepared and distributed a final report on the test-retest reliability of the Common Protocol, which was subsequently revised and published (Salyers and others, 2001).

At the request of the government program director, the coordinating center contracted with one of the PANSS creators to review videotaped PANSS assessments conducted at EIDP sites in order to develop gold standard PANSS ratings. On a monthly basis, the coordinating center distributed these tapes to each site, where interviewers scored them and submitted their ratings to the coordinating center, which conducted interrater reliability analysis and distributed reports summarizing each site's level of agreement and disagreement on symptom ratings, along with cross-site reliability results. All PANSS interviewers then participated with the scale's author in quarterly recalibration teleconference calls, at which interrater reliability results were reviewed, ratings were compared to the gold standard, and refresher training was conducted. In the months between teleconference calls, coordinating center staff collected, analyzed, and distributed monthly comparisons of gold standard PANSS ratings with site interviewers' ratings. The PANSS recalibration conference calls and interrater reliability analyses continued throughout the data collection period of the study.

Other Protocols. To develop service utilization measures, the coordinating center reviewed the service tracking procedures of each site to determine common service categories among treatment and control conditions and common service category definitions across sites. Working with steering committee members, coordinating center staff developed a protocol for service tracking procedures, data collection, and transfer of service data to the coordinating center. The coordinating center also convened a five-member cost panel and disseminated information packets to panel members, including site intervention summaries, site service tracking procedures, and cost analysis goals outlined in the original request for applications and in the coordinating center proposal. Cost panel members attended a steering committee meeting to discuss cost analysis plans and issues.

To ensure efficient and effective communication among the many EIDP project researchers, coordinating center staff assessed sites' Internet capabilities and hardware configurations. Technical assistance was delivered to project Internet users as required, successfully linking over fifty members of the steering committee and their associates to EIDP's electronic listserv, named empdemo. Once the link was established, a great deal of project discussions and decision making through consensus and voting took place on this listserv, which has been used throughout the project.

Study Implementation and Management

By the beginning of the second year, sites were preparing to enter the field and begin data collection. At the request of the government program director, the coordinating center began conducting ongoing monthly update calls with each of the site principal investigators to assess progress and note problems and developments. Information from these calls was summarized in monthly reports, including information about staff recruitment and retention, as well as research subject enrollment and study attrition. These reports were used in overall program management by the federal program director and in individual site management by the principal investigators.

In order to establish successful data transfer, computer programs were developed to check for outliers and logical inconsistencies. Data from sites were checked for problems and then returned to sites with outliers, invalid values, and logical inconsistencies flagged. The coordinating center received corrected data files back from sites and merged the resulting data into cross-site databases. Attention was focused on preliminary analyses of common protocol data concerning characteristics of study participants, equivalence of samples across study conditions within each project, preliminary employment outcome data, and preliminary service utilization data.

At the request of the government program director, the coordinating center surveyed sites to determine which sites were using fidelity measures for already established models such as the International Center for Clubhouse Development (ICCD), Program of Assertive Community Treatment (PACT), or Individual Placement and Support. As a result of this survey, the steering committee voted to develop a cross-program measure to collect information about the vocational models in use across all sites, regardless of whether they were using a previously developed fidelity scale. Working collaboratively with steering committee members, the coordinating center developed and helped pilot-test the Cross-Site Program Measure, designed so that all sites could be compared on a number of features, including staff composition and qualifications, caseload size and composition, the vocational rehabilitation approach underlying each service delivery model (that is, place-train versus train-place), the degree of consumer program involvement and governance, and the extent to which the vocational intervention was embedded in an auspice agency as well as the nature of that parent agency. This measure was developed during a series of conference calls that involved all sites, the coordinating center, the consumer representative, and the government program director. After the measure was finalized, the coordinating center prepared an administration manual for this measure and collected data on each of the seventeen conditions (seven EIDP sites had an experimental and control condition, and the eighth site had an experimental and two control conditions).

With the projects under way and data collection ongoing, supplemental funding was obtained from the Social Security Administration and other federal sources for the sites to develop and implement additional projects.

The coordinating center began a substudy of EIDP participants' personal economic situations, called the Personal Economy Survey. Working with the EIDP economist consultants, the coordinating center developed a separate protocol designed to capture detailed information about sources and amounts of monthly earned and unearned income, expenditures, assets, benefits and entitlements, and Supplemental Security Income/Social Security Disability Insurance histories. Individual sites also engaged in substudies, such as one site's assessment of consumer satisfaction through focus groups convened by consumer researchers, another site's ethnography of consumers' employment experiences, and a survey of employer attitudes and experiences at a third site.

In the fifth project year, two additional steering committee subcommittees were formed to advance the analytic work of the multisite study: the vocational outcomes subcommittee and the services subcommittee. The vocational outcomes subcommittee discussed and operationalized the major dependent variables of the cross-site analysis, including employment status, supported employment, competitive employment, job tenure, and amount of money earned. The services subcommittee worked on resolving a series of issues regarding how program services would be classified across programs and treated analytically. Because data collection continued throughout the entire fifth year of the project, it was necessary to extend activities into a sixth year, using carry-forward funds and some supplemental monies. During this sixth year, the coordinating center convened a number of work groups to guide the development of data analysis strategies to test the major EIDP research questions. These work groups, composed of steering committee members and members of the consumer assembly, advise the coordinating center on the types of data analyses appropriate for addressing the research questions posed by the original project request for applications.

Other important components include the development of a publication policy, power analysis recalculations necessitated by changes in subject recruitment and retention, Spanish-language translation of instruments, and the development of project and program logic models.

Knowledge Dissemination Activities

In response to the application phase of the KDA agenda, an impressive amount and variety of knowledge dissemination activities occurred throughout the project funding period, including oral and written presentations of EIDP findings, as well as technical assistance to consumers, advocates, policymakers, federal agencies, and the field at large. Steering committee members and coordinating center staff have presented numerous papers, plenary addresses, and keynote speeches and have participated in panels and employment tracks at national conferences, workshops, symposia, grand rounds, and trainings that featured information about EIDP. In addition, findings have been shared at conferences that focused on disabilities and were convened by federally funded rehabilitation research and training centers. Presentations also have been made at conferences organized by mental health consumers and family members, such as the annual Alternatives conference and the annual convention of the National Alliance for the Mentally Ill.

Dissemination also has involved work with the media. For example, research results regarding employment among homeless people with severe mental illness were provided to the editor of a Toronto-based newsletter, the *Journal of Addiction and Mental Health,* which is distributed throughout Canada. EIDP has been the subject of coverage by such newspapers as the *Fort Worth Star-Telegram,* the *Bowling Green Sentinel-Tribune,* and the *Washington Post.*

Early Impact of EIDP. On passage of the Ticket to Work and Work Incentives Improvement Act by Congress, which enables people with disabilities to enter the workforce without losing Medicaid and Medicare coverage, CMHS saw a tremendous opportunity for the early results of EIDP to affect the way the law would be implemented. Government program directors acted as liaisons between the study and the Social Security Administration, providing information on participant outcomes and process that informed policy development regarding that legislation. The coordinating center also worked with the steering committee to coordinate EIDP consumer participation in a special meeting of the Presidential Task Force on Employment of Adults with Disabilities, at which the task force presented its first-year report to Vice President Al Gore. EIDP findings were presented at the first White House Conference on Mental Health, convened by President Bill Clinton, and at a CMHS-sponsored employment summit, entitled "Hand in Hand," attended by employers, consumers, policymakers, and members of the House and Senate. A variety of federal agencies have received technical assistance, including the Center for Substance Abuse Treatment, the Center for Substance Abuse Prevention, the National Institute of Mental Health, the National Institute on Disability and Rehabilitation Research, the General Accounting Office, the Social Security Administration, the Department of Labor, and the Department of Veterans Affairs.

Web-Based Information. The EIDP Web site (www.psych.uic.edu/eidp) was developed collaboratively by the coordinating center and the steering committee to provide access to information about the ongoing activities of the multisite program, the eight individual sites, and the coordinating center. The Web site provides a comprehensive summary of the background and purpose of EIDP, the vocational rehabilitation models included in the program, contact information (electronic links as well as postal addresses and telephone contact information) for point-of-contact staff at the eight sites, the coordinating center, CMHS, the consumer representatives, and senior program consultants. A section on preliminary findings presents information on the characteristics of EIDP participants, as well as early results regarding employment outcomes and features of jobs held by EIDP participants, such as the amount of money earned, hours worked, and job tenure. A section describing EIDP products and activities is updated quarterly.

Site users may download copies of the EIDP Common Protocol, Employment Tracking Forms, the Common Protocol Documentation Manual, the Common Service Categories and Definitions, the Personal Economy Substudy Survey and Interviewer Guide, and the Cross-Site Program Measure.

Meeting Challenges Collaboratively

EIDP encountered a number of challenges that had to be surmounted for the study to be successful, and the initiative's collaborative structure of steering committee guidance and coordinating center activities proved equal to the task. The context of federal research, being a mix of science and established order, necessitated a gradual introduction of the ideal design. Projects selected for funding did not necessarily integrate to create an ideal multisite study. For example, one site's vocational service delivery model was designed for clients who entered the program already employed, whereas all other sites recruited nonworking participants. In the cross-site analysis, it was necessary to eliminate study participants who were employed at intake, as well as those who were assigned to one of the control groups at the site that used two control conditions; this lowered the sample size and statistical power of the entire study. Another challenge was that some projects' control conditions consisted of no service or service as usual, whereas other projects tested two viable models. This departure from a no-treatment, randomized clinical trials design created data analysis challenges necessitating steering committee consultation with a team of biostatisticians who have expertise in multilevel, multivariable analysis.

Although all projects consisted of some type of supported employment, service delivery models tested in the experimental conditions varied widely; this variation in service approach introduced a certain amount of conceptual noise that would not have existed if all projects tested the same vocational model. Some sites tested preexisting vocational rehabilitation models, and others created models of service delivery specially developed for the study. The fact that no fidelity measures existed for the newly developed models was problematic, as was the fact that some models were not fully operational during the early phases of data gathering. Moreover, during part of the study period, no agreed-on fidelity measures existed for some of the already developed models, such as PACT or the ICCD Clubhouse model. This made it difficult to assess fidelity over time to determine whether sites were actually delivering services according to the models they purported to be following. Steering committee members met this challenge by working collaboratively with the coordinating center to develop, field-test, and collect data using the EIDP Cross-Site Program Measure (available to other researchers and service providers on the EIDP Web site).

Another challenge was the fact that some site principal investigators had doubts about the requirements and viability of the multisite study design. For example, some principal investigators questioned the wisdom of data submission to the coordinating center on a quarterly basis. Other projects initially resented the data checks that the coordinating center performed and were slow to respond to reports indicating that their data were inaccurate or otherwise inadequate. Over time, however, it became clear that the massive amount and complexity of the EIDP database required this level of monitoring and that the steering committee and coordinating center, working together, could create a unique longitudinal data resource that would be one of the first of its kind, with implications and uses far beyond the research questions posed in the original request for applications.

The maintenance of interrater reliability both within and across sites was necessitated by the challenging nature of psychiatric symptom measurement that the steering committee decided to adopt as part of the common protocol. Because the degree of symptomatology was considered an important independent variable that the group wished to measure accurately, interviewers were trained in conducting PANSS, and this assessment was administered in a consistent, reliable way over time and across sites; as staff turnover occurred, additional training was required. Again, sites, the government project officer, and coordinating center staff met this challenge by developing and cooperating in an ongoing plan that resulted in high levels of intra- and intersite reliability and a unique opportunity to understand the interplay of psychiatric symptomatology and vocational outcomes.

The EIDP initiative faced a series of logistical challenges. Two separate shutdowns of the federal government occurred during the first year of the program, delaying the processing of paperwork and limiting the availability of federal personnel. This was especially problematic given that multisite studies typically require substantial forward momentum in their early phases, especially during the period of Common Protocol development and testing. Individual sites experienced unforeseen difficulties (one managed care provider entity went bankrupt, another program lost its executive director and the replacement was far less enthusiastic about study participation, and another site's principal investigator resigned during the course of the study and was replaced with a new investigator). Data analysis at all sites continued well past projected target dates, into the study's sixth year. Although these are problems common to all research projects, the sheer number of sites and conditions magnified the degree of difficulty that was presented to the program as a whole. The program also experienced a change in government program director twice during the course of the study, which introduced some uncertainty given the importance of that role in this particular multisite. Although the new CMHS staff proved to be knowledgeable and quick to learn about the study and how it functioned, EIDP's complexity made this a daunting task for replacements. But, again, the structure of the steering committee maintained the project's institutional memory throughout these various structural changes, and the coordinating center provided documentation for hundreds of steering committee decisions in its detailed minutes and tape recordings of all meetings and teleconferences, as well as archived empdemo listserv communications.

Looking Back at Lessons Learned

The major lesson learned from EIDP is that close and effective collaboration between a steering committee and coordinating center is crucial to the success of multisite projects because of the multitude of activities that must be undertaken to ensure the success of such a complex endeavor. Examples of activities enhanced by this collaboration include facilitating the participation of consumers in all phases of the research process, particularly the end stages of data analysis and interpretation. Other important collaborative tasks include ensuring validity and reliability of the research measures through careful monitoring and calibration, as well as maximizing homogeneity of data collection procedures through the creation of protocol documentation and immediate resolution of field-based problems. Another collaborative imperative is the coordination of intraprogram communication through frequent and regular face-to-face meetings (the coordinating center convened sixteen separate meetings of the steering committee in six states over five years), operation of an Internet listserv, and dissemination of various written documents and audiovisual materials. Another important task enriched by the collaboration of the steering committee and coordinating center was the construction and management of the complex EIDP database, requiring implementation of and cooperation with extensive computerized data checks, followed by data cleaning and resubmission procedures.

The close collaboration between the steering committee and coordinating center facilitated other collaborative efforts that were beneficial to the multisite project. Consultation from experts external to EIDP in a variety of areas was needed, and the professional relationships between EIDP researchers and their colleagues outside the study provided a rich pool of experts on which the project could draw. For example, scale authors were available for training and ongoing consultation, biostatistical experts were recruited to help resolve thorny statistical challenges, major figures in qualitative research provided workshops and ongoing consultation, and subcontracts for external fidelity analyses and consultation with mental health services economists were successfully executed. The critical role that the federal program director played in these collaborations is another important lesson learned in EIDP. This person was essential to ensure policy relevance of the findings, liaison with SAMHSA and other federal agencies, and provide management oversight to help the project stay on track and move forward.

Finally, maintaining the morale and collaborative spirit of such a challenging undertaking is an often overlooked, underappreciated responsibility that all must share. At every steering committee meeting, an effort was made to ensure opportunities for informal interpersonal contact, usually at a group dinner held on the first night of the meeting. These meals were often organized by the site hosting the meeting, adding some fun and local interest to the event. In addition, the coordinating center made every effort to make steering committee members comfortable during meetings, from accommodating locations and special requests to small jokes or candies provided throughout the long meeting days. Steering committee members' professional accomplishments or personal milestones were lauded during meetings, whenever possible and appropriate, adding to the feeling of camaraderie. Important mentorship and a sympathetic ear provided by the government program director also contributed to the program's esprit de corps. These efforts made at emphasizing extensive interpersonal contact created a strong group feeling for the steering committee, which survived the turnover of individual members.

The payback for these efforts comes when one compares the power of a prospective, well-executed multisite study with what can be learned from a set of individual, stand-alone studies compared on an ex post facto basis. There are many advantages to collecting data from a large number of participants, using standardized protocols that have been administered in a uniform manner and monitored for data accuracy and consistency. These include the ability to conduct a wide range of statistical analyses that are far more powerful and informative than the typical meta-analytic approaches used to compare stand-alone studies. Another advantage is the creation of a large, well-documented database that can be used to address questions beyond those that were the original focus of the initiative. Related to this is the opportunity presented by multisite studies to increase the relevance of study findings by combining multiple perspectives (such as research, government, consumer, and family) in the design and conduct of the inquiry.

Conclusion

Close and effective collaboration among the various parties to the EIDP endeavor was essential to the study's success. This chapter has described numerous ways in which the coordinating center and steering committee worked together to identify and overcome the many evaluation challenges that confront large and complex research undertakings. Although it is inevitable that each party to a multisite study is committed to accomplishing unique and sometimes conflicting aims, in the end, a sense of common purpose and spirit of compromise formed the foundation of both study rigor and the relevance of research results.

References

Cook, J. A. "Research on Psychosocial Rehabilitation Services for Persons with Psychiatric Disabilities." *Psychotherapy and Rehabilitation Research Bulletin*, 1995, 4, 5–11.

Cook, J. A., and Razzano, L. A. "Vocational Rehabilitation for Persons with Schizophrenia: Recent Research and Implications for Practice." *Schizophrenia Bulletin,* 2000, *26,* 87–103.

Kay, S. R., Opler, L. A., and Fishbein, A. *Positive and Negative Syndrome Scale (PANSS) Manual.* North Tonawanda, N.Y.: Multi-Health Systems, 1986.

Salyers, M. P., and others. "Reliability of Instruments in a Cooperative, Multisite Study: Employment Intervention Demonstration Program." *Mental Health Services Research,* 2001, *3,* 129–140.

JUDITH A. COOK *is principal investigator of the Employment Intervention Demonstration Program coordinating center and professor in the Department of Psychiatry at the University of Illinois at Chicago.*

MARTHA ANN CAREY, *a social psychologist, was the first program director of the Employment Intervention Demonstration Program. She is now with the National Institute of Mental Health, National Institutes of Health, Bethesda, Maryland.*

LISA A. RAZZANO *is project director of the Employment Intervention Demonstration Program coordinating center and assistant professor in the Department of Psychiatry at the University of Illinois at Chicago.*

JANE BURKE *is project manager of the Employment Intervention Demonstration Program coordinating center and a research analyst in the Department of Psychiatry at the University of Illinois at Chicago.*

CRYSTAL R. BLYLER *is a social science analyst with the Center for Mental Health Services and has served as the government project officer for and federal representative to the Employment Intervention Demonstration Program steering committee since 1998.*

4

This chapter describes a technique based on meta-analysis for analyzing data from multisite studies.

A Prospective Meta-Analytic Approach in a Multisite Study of Homelessness Prevention

Steven Banks, Gregory J. McHugo, Valerie Williams, Robert E. Drake, Marybeth Shinn

In the past decade, there has been a proliferation of federally funded multisite studies. Kraemer (2000) described different types of multisite studies, which range from studies with a single intervention, research protocol, and subject population to studies that use a common data-gathering protocol but differ in intervention composition and subject population. She called these "multiple collaborating single-site randomized clinical trials" (p. 533). Such was the situation facing our project, and thus, we implemented an analytic method that was appropriate for this type of multisite study.

This research is a product of the collaborative effort of the Analysis and Taxonomy Subcommittees of the Collaborative Program to Prevent Homelessness. We gratefully acknowledge the contributions of the investigators: Sara Asmussen, John Brekke, Colleen Clark, Kendon Conrad, Kathleen Coughey, Patricia Hanrahan, Charles Reichardt, Alexander Rich, Joann Sacks, Stanley Sacks, Sam Tsemberis, Gregory Teague, and John Yagelka, as well as Lawrence Rickards, James Herrell, and Cheryl Gallagher of the Substance Abuse and Mental Health Services Administration (SAMHSA). Thanks also go to Pamela Robbins, Roumen Vesselinov, and William Shadish for their comments on an earlier version of this chapter.

This research was supported by grant no. 280–94–0008 from the Center for Substance Abuse Treatment and the Center for Mental Health Services, SAMHSA, U.S. Department of Health and Human Services. The views presented here are the authors' and do not necessarily represent the official policy or position of SAMHSA.

Our approach can be described as a prospective meta-analysis because it employs meta-analytic methods that are usually used to summarize published research in conjunction with the hypothetico-deductive approach to analyzing clinical trials. These techniques offer a wide range of accessibility to audiences and an ease of testing various alternative hypotheses, making them potentially applicable to a variety of multisite evaluations. In this chapter, we provide the scientific rationale for the analytic strategy, the statistical formulas to perform the analysis, and an example from a multisite study evaluating the effectiveness of various treatment interventions to prevent homelessness.

When a meta-analysis of published results is performed, the review's purpose and research questions are developed. Published results are then selected by applying specified procedures for locating studies that meet explicit criteria for inclusion in the analysis. Data are collected from studies by coding study features according to the objectives of the review and as checks on threats to validity, as well as by transforming study outcomes into a common metric so they can be combined and compared. The typical metric is the effect size, defined as the standardized difference in outcome between the average study participant who received a treatment and the average participant who did not (or who received a different level of treatment). Finally, statistical procedures are used to investigate relationships among study characteristics and findings. When a meta-analytic approach is used to analyze data from a multisite study, many of the central features of traditional meta-analysis, such as computation of a study-specific effect size and exploration of relationships among study characteristics and findings, remain integral.

Study Description

In 1996, the Center for Mental Health Services (CMHS) and the Center for Substance Abuse Treatment (CSAT) of the Substance Abuse and Mental Health Services Administration (SAMHSA) launched a three-year cooperative agreement, the Collaborative Program to Prevent Homelessness (CPPH), to evaluate the effectiveness of various interventions in eight sites across the United States (Rickards and others, 1999). This study targeted persons with psychiatric and substance use disorders who were formerly homeless or at risk of homelessness and who were engaged with the mental health or substance abuse treatment systems. Eight sites (Chicago, Denver, Los Angeles, Tampa/St. Petersburg, New York City, Philadelphia [two sites], and Washington, D.C.) were selected because they represented combinations of mental health and substance abuse services with four strategies for homelessness prevention: supported housing, residential treatment, family support and respite, and representative payee and money management. Across the sites, the population considered to be at risk varied in the extent and severity of current and lifetime homelessness, mental illness, and substance abuse. Six sites were mental health programs, and two were primarily substance abuse treatment programs. (For a detailed description of the participating sites and CPPH, see Rickards and others, 1999.)

Challenges and Resolutions to the CPPH Cross-Site Analysis

Although the CPPH sites were diverse in their settings and approaches, they had common components: (1) a connection to, or provision of, a range of affordable, safe housing options, (2) flexible case management services of varying intensity, (3) linkages to mental health or substance abuse treatment, (4) money management, and (5) a range of community support services. Differences among the interventions centered on the quantity of services provided within the five key components and the range of outreach and enrollment procedures.

The settings in which outreach and recruitment were conducted, as well as the enrollment procedures used, covered various points of entry into the service system, from street outreach to community mental health agencies. There are two important implications of these differences. First, participants recruited into the intervention settings were at different points along the homeless continuum, and these points of entry mirrored risk factors that have been identified as pathways to homelessness. Some participants were homeless at the time of recruitment, whereas others may have been actively engaged in the treatment system but lacking the appropriate supports needed to maintain housing. Second, participants represented different populations (for example, mothers with children in therapeutic communities, users of detoxification facilities, people living on the streets) that did not simply reflect differences in stage of homelessness.

Additional site differences posed challenges for the development of a cross-site analytic framework. First, sites used different methods for assigning participants to treatment (that is, intervention programs) and comparison groups. Some sites used random assignment, and others used a quasi-experimental design with naturally formed groups. Second, differences in intervention and comparison programs exist across sites; that is, the comparison group at one site may have been similar to the intervention group at another site. To address this difference in study groups across sites, we developed and used a set of program-level contrasts to classify the sites.

Program-level data were collected on the intervention components at each site in the domains of housing, case management, and other services and treatment foci. This information was obtained with the Program Characteristics Measure (PCM) (Teague and others, 2000; Policy Research Associates, 2001), which was completed for each of the study groups at all sites, allowing comparisons to be made between intervention and comparison group scores on items in the three overarching domains. Each PCM item was rated on a scale from 1 to 5. A rating of 1 indicated that the component was not characteristic of the program, whereas a 5 meant that the component was very characteristic of the program. For example, the first item in the housing domain, "control of housing stock," was defined as "the agency controls access to housing so that it can guarantee availability to study participants." A score of 1 on this item indicated that the agency had no control over housing stock, and a score of 5 meant that an agency could guarantee access to respondents (that is, the agency owned all buildings in which housing was located or had vouchers for all housing units offered to participants). Teague and others (2000) describe the development and use of PCM in the CPPH cross-site analysis.

Contrast scores on each PCM item were calculated by subtracting the score for each site's comparison group from the score for that site's intervention group. Principal investigators agreed that a contrast score of 2 or more (absolute value) represented the cutoff for determining whether there was a meaningful difference between the two study groups at each site. Thus, a site would be considered to have no contrast on a PCM item if both intervention and comparison groups scored high on the item or if both groups scored low; that is, a contrast is a function not of the experimental treatment but of the difference between the experimental and comparison conditions at a particular site.

The Prospective Meta-Analytic Method

The prospective meta-analytic approach employed five sequential steps, all based on the calculation of site-level effect sizes. First, we examined the overall difference between the intervention and comparison groups across sites, using a meta-analytic approach to summarize and weight data from each of the sites. Second, we examined whether there was significant heterogeneity of effect sizes across sites. Third, given heterogeneity, we attempted to model it using a priori contrasts on the specific components of interventions at the different sites. Fourth, given a contrast accounting for significant variance, we examined the sensitivity of the test to the inclusion of particular sites. Confidence increases if the results are not dependent on the inclusion of particular sites in the overall analysis. Finally, we tested moderators to determine whether conclusions held across demographic groups and groups that differed on baseline characteristics relevant to the interventions. This last step did not depend on the previous ones; for example, moderating effects can be tested whether an overall effect is found or is homogeneous.

The prospective component of this analytic strategy borrows heavily from randomized clinical trial literature. The first prospective decision was to analyze the data in an intent-to-treat model; that is, an individual initially in the intervention group (whether randomized or self-selected) is considered in this group regardless of whether he or she makes use of the intervention services. This preserves the design features of a randomized study. A second decision was to identify a small set of primary outcome measures for analysis of the intervention effect. If there is a significant overall intervention effect or significant intervention effect heterogeneity, additional analyses can be performed without controlling for the multiplicity of statistical tests (Snedecor and Cochran, 1980). If significant differences exist among the effects across the sites, then these differences need to be modeled with program-level factors. Furthermore, the sensitivity of the results should be examined to see if particular sites dominate the conclusions (Greenhouse and Iyengar, 1994). Third, these program-level factors need to be identified in advance of examining the outcomes. Fourth, potential participant-level moderator variables should be identified before the analyses of the outcomes. The a priori nature of the decisions increases the statistical interpretability of the resulting p values. All of these a priori steps were taken in the multisite analysis outlined here and justify describing the meta-analysis as prospective.

Computing Site-Specific Effect Sizes

The computation of an effect size for each project is an essential component of a prospective meta-analytic approach. In our study, the choice of a measure of effect size for each outcome variable at each study site depended on whether there were significant differences between intervention and comparison groups at baseline. When significant differences did not exist, analysis of covariance (ANCOVA) was used to generate the information for computing the effect size (see formula 1 in the chapter technical appendix). Groups were presumed to come from the same population, and the introduction of the covariate simply increased the precision of the estimate.

When a site's study groups were not equivalent on the outcome measure of interest at baseline, a standardized mean difference was used to compute an effect size (see formula 2 in the technical appendix). In this situation, ANCOVA can introduce bias, and regression of each group to its respective population mean can be mistakenly interpreted as an effect of treatment—the so-called Lord's Paradox (Lord, 1967).

Where samples are small, measures of effect size are upwardly biased and can be corrected with a simple formula (see formula 3 in the technical appendix). This adjustment reduces the effect size for studies with seventy-eight or more subjects by less than 1 percent.

Computing a Mean Effect Size

Once an effect size is calculated for each project, an estimate of the average effect across all sites is computed. Because sites have different numbers of subjects, we computed a weighted mean effect size (see formula 4 in the technical appendix).

Having computed the mean effect size and its variability, we can test the hypothesis that the mean effect size equals zero. This test is the first of several that form the logical hierarchy in the prospective meta-analysis. For this hypothesis to be tested, the 95 percent confidence interval is formed around the mean effect size (see formula 5 in the technical appendix). If the confidence interval includes zero, we cannot demonstrate any overall effect of the interventions across all sites. If the confidence interval does not include zero, the mean effect size is considered to be different from zero. Two questions then arise. First, how big is the effect? Cohen (1977) and Lipsey (1990) have provided rules for labeling effect sizes as small, medium, and large. The second question concerning the variability among the site effect sizes is discussed in the next section.

For clarity, effect sizes can be converted back into the scale of the outcome variable. In CPPH, the primary outcome variables were measures of time in various residential settings, so effect sizes were converted back into days. Days were calculated by multiplying the mean effect size by the median standard deviation across the sites to yield the difference in the proportion of days. We then multiplied this quantity by 180, the approximate number of days in a six-month period.

Assessing Heterogeneity of Effect Sizes Among the Sites

Assessing the variability of effect sizes is of substantial scientific interest. To the extent that there is significant heterogeneity among the effect sizes, the variability will be modeled with the program-level variables. In contrast, if the effect sizes appear homogeneous, the analysis may proceed to the examination of moderator variables. To assess the degree of heterogeneity among a group of effect sizes, we used a technique described by Hedges and Olkin (1985). This technique is similar to the analysis of variance and produces a chi-square statistic with the number of degrees of freedom equal to one less than the number of sites being analyzed (see formula 6 in the technical appendix). A significant chi-square statistic indicates that significant heterogeneity exists among the effect sizes, and interest turns to understanding the reason.

Modeling the Heterogeneity of Effect Sizes

The Hedges and Olkin (1985) method of examining heterogeneity can also be used to test factors associated with the heterogeneity. The approach partitions the total heterogeneity into components explained by a contrast variable and a pooled residual within-groups component. With the CPPH example, the test of total heterogeneity among the eight sites' effect sizes produced a chi-square with seven degrees of freedom. If significant variation is observed, the sites can be disaggregated into two clusters, based on a program-level factor: those with a contrast and those with no contrast. This procedure is repeated first using only sites with a contrast and again using sites with no contrast. For example, if there are five sites with a contrast and three with no contrast, the chi-square statistic for sites with a contrast will have four degrees of freedom, whereas the chi-square for sites with no contrast will have two degrees of freedom. The theory associated with partitioning of chi-square statistics indicates that

> Total heterogeneity = Heterogeneity within no-contrast group + heterogeneity within high-contrast group + difference between high- and no-contrast groups

In this formula, the last term is also a chi-square statistic with one degree of freedom. If this term is significant, the effect of the intervention differs significantly between the contrast and no-contrast sites. The other two chi-square statistics can be tested separately or pooled to test whether significant heterogeneity remains after controlling for this single program-level factor.

Where a significant effect size was observed for a cluster of sites and the heterogeneity within that cluster was significant, sensitivity analyses were conducted to determine whether the effect was the consequence of a single project (Greenhouse and Iyengar, 1994). There are a number of ways to accomplish this test of sensitivity. One is to remove each site's effect size, one at a time, from the analysis and to repeat the computations. With this approach, the power of the multisite analysis is reduced, as computations are now on seven sites, with fewer cases. A second method is to replace the effect size for the site with the largest impact with the next largest effect size observed. This serves to pull the largest effect size toward the mean of the other sites in its cluster. If reanalysis indicates that the significant effect is maintained, confidence in its robustness increases.

The extent to which respondent characteristics moderated site-level effects can also be examined with the partitioning of a chi-square approach. For CPPH, we used a set of participant-level covariates (gender, for example) as a method to reduce further the heterogeneity of effects observed and determine whether programs were differentially successful for individuals with particular characteristics. For example, the effect of gender, contrast, and a gender-by-contrast interaction could all be estimated with the partitioned chi-squares.

The sensitivity, or robustness, of these analyses is also of interest. A weaker test of robustness was employed by removing individual sites and determining whether there was a change in the direction of the interaction, computed as the difference score between the two covariate groups (males versus females, for example) across the two clusters.

Results Using a Single Outcome Variable

In this section, we use one of the primary outcome measures, stable housing, to illustrate the prospective meta-analytic method. Stable housing was computed from the Residential Follow-Back Calendar data as described in more detail elsewhere (Policy Research Associates, 2001). Days in stable housing is the sum of the days spent during the interview period in the respondent's own single room occupancy (SRO) unit, apartment or house, a supportive SRO, long-term transitional housing program or group home, or the apartment or house (long term) of the respondent's parent or guardian or someone else. Because interview periods varied in duration, we calculated the proportion of days in these settings in the interview period.

In general, clients in the comparison groups across the sites showed significant improvement in the proportion of days stably housed, comparing the first six months in the study period to the six months before enrollment in the study (Wilcoxon signed rank test, $p < .05$). For an intervention to produce a positive effect, improvement in the intervention group must exceed that in the comparison group. Tables 4.1 and 4.2 present the cross-site results for stable housing during the period from baseline to six-month follow-up. The 95 percent confidence interval in Table 4.2 does not include zero, which means that the change in stable housing represents a significant improvement in the intervention programs relative to the comparison programs. Across all sites, the advantage of the intervention groups over the comparison groups was approximately twelve additional days in stable housing. The substantial degree of heterogeneity among the sites' effect sizes (chi-square value in Table 4.2) means that the distribution of effect sizes for stable housing does not estimate a common population mean effect size. In other words, all sites' interventions did not exhibit the same differential effect on stable housing relative to their comparison conditions. After finding that the sites' effect sizes were not homogeneous, we continued to assume a fixed effects model with the added assumption that the excess variability was due to identifiable differences between the sites. However, a random effects model could have been followed with this same general approach (Lipsey and Wilson, 2001).

The excess variability observed across the eight sites was modeled with the "control of housing stock" program-level factor. Table 4.3 shows the

Table 4.1. Sample and Effect Sizes by Site for the Stable Housing Measure at Six-Month Follow-Up

	N	Effect Size
1	131	.22
2	196	1.60
3	106	− .86[a]
4	78	− .28
5	113	.14
6	68	.70
7	93	− .18
8	259	− .04

[a]Mean difference effect size computed owing to nonequivalence on this measure at baseline.

Table 4.2. Cross-Site Results for the Stable Housing at Six-Month Follow-Up

Proportion of Time Stably Housed	Mean Adjusted Effect Size Across Eight Sites	Confidence Interval (95% CI)	Days per Six Months	Within-Group Heterogeneity
Baseline to six-month follow-up	.22	(.09 − .34)	12	$\chi^2 = 111.75$[a] (df = 7)

[a]$p < .001$. There is substantial variability across the sites. This variation is maintained even when the most influential effect size is replaced by the next largest effect size (for example, when the effect size of project 2 was replaced by the effect size of project 6).

results for stable housing of stratifying the sites by the presence or absence of a contrast on this program-level factor. The contrast group (projects 1, 2, 5, and 6) showed a larger overall effect than the no-contrast group (projects 3, 4, 7, and 8) ($\chi^2 = 54.56$, df = 1). On average, members of the intervention groups in sites with contrasts on control of housing stock were stably housed for an additional forty days over the six-month period between baseline and six months, relative to members of the comparison groups in the same sites. Although control of housing stock explained a significant portion of the variability observed among the effect sizes, a significant amount of variance remained in both of the clusters after stratification, as indicated by the chi-square values for within-cluster heterogeneity in Table 4.3. Substantially more variability was observed in the contrast cluster than in the no-contrast cluster. In this example, examination of the within-cluster heterogeneity was not possible because of the small number of sites, but in principle, such further examination is possible and would be warranted if there was a basis for another level of clustering.

With the sensitivity analysis, we replaced the largest effect size in the contrast group (1.60) with the next largest effect size (.70) and repeated the analysis. The difference between intervention and comparison groups in the proportion of days in stable housing in the contrast cluster remained

Table 4.3. Difference in Stable Housing Between Clusters of Sites Based on Control of Housing Stock

Proportion of Time Stably Housed	Contrast on Control of Housing Stock			No Contrast on Control of Housing Stock			
	Effect Size (95% CI)	Days per Six Months	Within-Cluster Heterogeneity	Effect Size (95% CI)	Days per Six Months	Within-Cluster Heterogeneity	Significance of Contrast
Baseline versus six-month follow-up	.72 (.53 − .90)	40	$\chi^2 = 45.67$** (df=3)	− .25 (−.43 − .07)	−14	$\chi^2 = 11.52$* (df=3)	$\chi^2 = 54.56$** (df=1)

*$p < .05$. **$p < .01$.

significant, albeit smaller (twenty days as opposed to forty days in Table 4.3). Thus, the conclusion about the importance of control of housing stock for increasing time in stable housing did not depend on just one site.

As another means to model the remaining heterogeneity among the effect sizes within the control of housing stock cluster, we examined age, gender, extent of lifetime homelessness, substance use, mental health symptomatology, and criminal activity as possible moderators of intervention effects. Only gender moderated the effects for control of housing stock, with this factor proving significantly more important for males than for females. The interaction was deemed robust because it remained on the same side of zero (although it did not retain significance) when each site in turn was removed from the analysis.

Lessons Learned

CPPH generated some important findings. In general, intervention programs produced a greater increase in the proportion of days in stable housing than did the comparison programs. Furthermore, there was significant heterogeneity among the sites, indicating that the effects of the interventions were not uniform. The four sites that had a contrast on the control of housing stock factor also had a larger mean effect size for days in stable housing than the four sites with no contrast on this factor. In addition, we tested several participant-level covariates as possible moderators of the effects within each control of housing stock cluster. Only gender proved significant, with the effect for control of housing stock larger for men than for women. (A more detailed presentation and discussion of these findings are available in the cross-site report: Policy Research Associates, 2001.)

Future studies may find the prospective meta-analytic framework more suitable for the analysis of multisite data than other methods, such as pooling the data or using hierarchical linear models. Factors to consider in making this choice include the extent of standardization of populations, interventions, setting characteristics (for example, ancillary services, organizational context), comparison conditions, and site-specific designs (for example, random assignment versus self-selection). Although suitable in virtually all cases, the prospective meta-analytic method may be the method of choice when there is a lack of standardization across sites on the factors given above. The focus of the prospective meta-analysis on the within-site effect sizes preserved site identity while allowing for the testing of multisite hypotheses.

For a meta-analysis to be prospective, a number of steps need to be taken up front. Given the decision to model the heterogeneity of the effect sizes across sites, the most important step is the elaboration and measurement of program-level factors that will be examined at the multisite level. This involves developing a taxonomy to characterize each site's intervention and comparison groups and assessing the contrast between the groups at each site on each factor in the taxonomy. The challenge is to identify a core set of program-level factors that captures variation among sites and divides them into roughly balanced clusters. Program-level factors on which very few or nearly all sites have a contrast cannot be tested effectively at the multisite level. Highly correlated factors may be combined or eliminated in order to arrive at a final number less than or equal to the degrees of freedom available to test for heterogeneity. Strategies for assessing site-level contrasts need to be developed early, so that appropriate data can be collected. Ratings of program fidelity provide data to use in deciding on the contrasts between intervention and comparison groups at each site. Participant self-reports of services used, provider logs of activity, and program management information systems are other sources of relevant data. Teague and others (2000) describe the process of developing and assessing the contrasts used in CPPH.

In addition to program-level factors that are based on within-site contrasts between study groups, it is also possible to consider factors based on identifiable differences among the sites. Site-level factors include contextual (urban versus rural sites) and methodological (random assignment versus self-selection) differences across sites that are hypothesized to moderate effect sizes. Program-level factors were primary in CPPH because they derive from experimental contrasts and thus enable causal inferences. Site-level factors are based on observation and lead to correlational inferences, although the computational procedures in the meta-analysis are identical.

Additional decisions that inform the prospective meta-analysis include choices of primary outcome measures and moderator variables. In CPPH, we chose seven outcome measures for the cross-site analysis; we presented the results for the proportion of time in stable housing. We limited the number of outcome variables to protect against inferential errors that result from many statistical tests. We also decided on a small set of participant-level variables to examine for moderator effects, both to limit inferential errors and to contain the conceptual scope of the cross-site analysis.

Other decisions that were made collectively before cross-site analyses concerned the site-level effect size and the sensitivity analyses. We decided to use the residualized effect size when the intervention and comparison groups were equivalent at baseline and the standardized mean difference when they were nonequivalent. Tests of the sensitivity of the results to the exclusion of particular sites provided an assessment of the robustness of the findings. This step is especially important when the number of sites is small, because one site can exert undue influence. The point in describing the preanalysis decision process is to underscore the cooperation and planning required to make the meta-analysis prospective. The CPPH steering committee spent a year preparing for the cross-site analyses so that we were ready to execute them as soon as the end-point data were available. This process educated participants, developed consensus for the approach, and reinforced the role that each site had in the multisite study. Because so much was decided beforehand, the analyses went very quickly, few decisions had to be made by the analysts, and the findings were communicated easily to investigators.

What are the advantages and disadvantages of the prospective meta-analytic approach over contemporary methods like hierarchical linear models (or other mixed-effects regression approaches) and structural equation models for the analysis of multisite data? Given the relative infancy of these methods, this question is difficult to answer until direct comparisons between them are made. In the case of CPPH, the answer is as much practical as it is technical. The prospective meta-analytic approach fit more closely with the mental models that participants had of the multisite study. Site identity was important, and the analysis had to preserve it in a transparent way. By basing the analysis on the site-level effect sizes, we focused on the site-by-treatment interaction, that is, on the differences among treatment effects across the eight sites. Differences among the sites at baseline or due to time alone were deemed secondary and were not part of the analysis plan.

The prospective meta-analytic method also enabled us to compute different forms of the effect size across the sites and to conduct appropriate sensitivity analyses. These steps would be more complicated and opaque with other statistical techniques. These other techniques (Haddock, Rindskopf, and Shadish, 1998) may produce more accurate estimates of variances, because of their use of the raw data and sophisticated computational algorithms, but the extent and importance of this advantage are not known.

One clear limitation of most multisite studies is the lack of statistical power to test hypotheses at the multisite level. With only eight sites in CPPH, the power to test program-level factors was minimal, as it would be with any other statistical approach. This lack of power may underidentify important program-level factors, but those found are likely to be robust. In CPPH, the control of housing stock explained variation in the effect sizes for residential outcomes across the sites, but other program-level factors did not. This effect withstood sensitivity tests, and it was further elaborated on by the interaction with gender. These significant effects emerged despite the lack of statistical power. One unanswered question concerns the credibility of findings that arise from multisite studies that employ a meta-analytic approach. How will scientists and policymakers view the key findings from CPPH? Do findings from a coordinated multisite study with a prospective meta-analysis deserve more consideration than findings from single-site studies and retrospective meta-analyses? The proliferation of multisite studies, especially into realms where conventional levels of standardization are not possible, will force examination of these questions in the coming years.

Conclusion

Making key analytic decisions prospectively and using an accessible approach can make the analysis of multisite data a more collaborative and productive process. The prospective meta-analytic approach is based on sound statistical methods and a clear conceptual framework. In multisite studies where there are specific features of design, measurement, or implementation that result in nonignorable differences among the sites, the prospective meta-analytic approach offers advantages over other approaches. The involvement of all CPPH investigators in decisions concerning the analysis and the simplicity and focus of the meta-analysis itself were important advantages of the approach and enhanced the overall quality of the multisite study.

Technical Appendix

All of the formulas presented here are provided in Hedges and Olkin (1985) and Lipsey and Wilson (2001).

Formula 1. To calculate the effect size with ANCOVA, we used the outcome measure at six months as the dependent variable. Study group, as an indicator variable B, and a covariate for the dependent measure at baseline were included in the model as predictor variables:

$$\text{Effect size} = \frac{\beta_{\text{studygroup}}}{\sqrt{MSE}}$$

The square root of the mean square error (MSE) is the best estimate of the pooled standard deviation (Rosenthal, 1994).

Formula 2. Raw difference effect sizes are computed by the following formula:

$$\text{Effect size} = \frac{\text{Mean change score}_{\text{int}} - \text{mean change score}_{\text{co}}}{s_p}$$

where *mean change score*$_{\text{int}}$ is the mean of the change scores for the intervention group, *mean change score*$_{\text{co}}$ is the mean of the change scores for the comparison group, and s_p is the pooled standard deviation of the change scores. The pooled standard deviation is calculated in the standard way.

Formula 3. The following formula adjusts for sample size:

$$\text{Adjusted effect size} = \left[1 - \frac{3}{4N - 9}\right]ES$$

where N is a study's total sample size and ES is the effect size.

Formula 4. Weighted mean effect sizes were computed with the following formula:

$$\text{Mean effect size} = \frac{\Sigma(w_i ES_i)}{\Sigma w_i}$$

where ES_i is the effect size for each study and w_i is the weight for each study. The weight is calculated as

$$w_i = \frac{1}{v_i}$$

where v_i is the variance of the effect size. The variance of the effect size is

$$ES_i = \frac{(n_{int})_i + (n_{co})_i}{(n_{int})_i(n_{co})_i} + \frac{ES_i^2}{2[(n_{int})_i + (n_{co})_i]}$$

where n_{int} is the size of the intervention group and n_{co} is the size of the comparison group in each project.

Formula 5. The 95 percent confidence interval is

$$\text{mean effect size}_{LL} = \text{mean effect size} - 1.96(\overline{se}_{\text{effect size}})$$

$$\text{mean effect size}_{UL} = \text{mean effect size} + 1.96(\overline{se}_{\text{effect size}})$$

where *mean effect sizes LL* and *UL* are the lower and upper limits of the confidence interval, respectively, and is the standard error of the mean effect size, computed as

$$\overline{se}_{\text{effect size}} = \sqrt{\frac{1}{\sum w_i}}$$

Formula 6. The heterogeneity, or dissimilarity, is

$$\text{Heterogeneity} = \sum wessq_i - \frac{(\sum wes_i)^2}{\sum w_i}$$

where $wessq_i = w_i(ES_i)^2$ and $wes_i = w_i(ES_i)$.

References

Cohen, J. *Statistical Power Analysis for the Behavioral Sciences.* (Rev. ed.) Orlando, Fla.: Academic Press, 1977.

Greenhouse, J. B., and Iyengar, S. "Sensitivity Analysis and Diagnostics." In H. Cooper and L. V. Hedges (Eds.), *The Handbook of Research Synthesis.* New York: Russell Sage Foundation, 1994.

Haddock, C. K., Rindskopf, D., and Shadish, W. R. "Using Odds Ratios as Effect Sizes for Meta-Analysis of Dichotomous Data: A Primer on Methods and Issues." *Psychological Methods,* 1998, 3, 339–353.

Hedges, L. V., and Olkin, I. *Statistical Methods for Meta-Analysis.* Orlando, Fla.: Academic Press, 1985.

Kraemer, H. C. "Pitfalls of Multisite Randomized Clinical Trials of Efficacy and Effectiveness." *Schizophrenia Bulletin,* 2000, 26, 533–541.

Lipsey, M. W. *Design Sensitivity: Statistical Power for Experimental Research.* Thousand Oaks, Calif.: Sage, 1990.

Lipsey, M. W., and Wilson, D. B. *Practical Meta-Analysis.* Thousand Oaks, Calif.: Sage, 2001.

Lord, F. M. "A Paradox in the Interpretation of Group Comparisons." *Psychological Bulletin,* 1967, 68, 304–305.

Policy Research Associates. *Final Report: Cross-Site Evaluation of the Collaborative Program to Prevent Homelessness.* Delmar, N.Y.: Policy Research Associates, 2001.

Rickards, L. D., and others. "Cooperative Agreements for CMHS/CSAT Collaborative Program to Prevent Homelessness: An Overview." *Alcoholism Treatment Quarterly,* 1999, *17,* 1–15.

Rosenthal, R. "Parametric Measures of Effect Size." In H. Cooper and L. V. Hedges (Eds.), *The Handbook of Research Synthesis.* New York: Russell Sage Foundation, 1994.

Snedecor, G. W., and Cochran, W. G. *Statistical Methods.* (7th ed.) Ames: Iowa State University Press, 1980.

Teague, G., and others. "Measurement of Interventions in a Multi-Site Study of Homelessness Prevention." Paper presented at the annual meeting of the American Public Health Association, Boston, Nov. 2000.

STEVEN BANKS *is research associate professor of psychiatry at the University of Massachusetts Medical School, Worcester.*

GREGORY J. MCHUGO *is research associate professor of psychiatry at Dartmouth College, Hanover, New Hampshire.*

VALERIE WILLIAMS *is a research associate with Policy Research Associates, Delmar, New York.*

ROBERT E. DRAKE *is professor of psychiatry at Dartmouth College, Hanover, New Hampshire.*

MARYBETH SHINN *is professor of psychology at New York University.*

5

The Center for Mental Health Services Housing Initiative illustrates the benefits of prior research, a phased approach, and strong collaboration in tackling difficult multisite issues.

A Multisite Evaluation of Supported Housing: Lessons Learned from Cross-Site Collaboration

Debra J. Rog, Frances L. Randolph

Much has been discussed in the previous chapters regarding the readiness of an intervention for a multisite study. Among the factors that affect readiness are how much previous research has been conducted and whether there is evidence of the efficacy of the treatment to submit it to a broader test of effectiveness. If a multisite evaluation is conducted on an ill-defined intervention or an emerging problem area (Edwards, 1987; Rog, 1994), the lack of a developed knowledge base challenges the sites' ability to follow uniform procedures in implementing the treatment and control conditions, defining and recruiting the study population, and even collecting core information.

In the housing arena for persons with serious mental illness, there has been considerable descriptive research over the past two decades on the types of housing provided and the needs and preferences of persons with mental illness (Rog, Holupka, and Brito, 1996). In addition, there have been efforts at developing a model of housing, called supported housing, that have captured the interests and support of consumers and many

This research was supported by grant no. 280–94–0008 from the Center for Substance Abuse Treatment and the Center for Mental Health Services, Substance Abuse and Mental Health Services Administration (SAMHSA), U.S. Department of Health and Human Services. The interpretations and conclusions contained in this article are the views of the authors and do not necessarily represent the position of the coordinating center, the study sites (Connecticut, Maricopa County, Massachusetts, upstate New York, New York City, and Oregon), the consumer advisory panel, or SAMHSA.

providers, though there has been no rigorous test of the model's effectiveness (Newman, 2001).

The research to date on housing provided the Center for Mental Health Services (CMHS) Housing Initiative with a sufficient foundation to mount a multisite study. Past work on the features of supported housing permitted the initiative to operationalize a very specific model of supported housing that could be examined with the same cross-site lens. In addition, despite the lack of prior effectiveness studies, the fact that supported housing had become so widespread and had presumed effectiveness suggested the need for an explicit, rigorous, multisite test of its actual effectiveness. A multisite study was viewed as an opportunity to accelerate the development of a knowledge base on the outcomes of this model for persons with serious mental illness.

In this chapter, we highlight some of the advantages of conducting a multisite study when the treatment condition has been the focus of much developmental work and prior investigation (though largely descriptive). In particular, we describe the importance of having the ability to prescribe a uniform model and how it can strengthen the cross-site analysis, reporting, and dissemination.

This chapter also illustrates the benefits of having a phased approach to multisite efforts. Because of the dynamic nature of housing and the exigencies in mounting a study in this area with this population, the federal government funded a two-phase evaluation approach, in which Phase I grantees completed process evaluations before competing for conducting Phase II outcome evaluations. Conducting process evaluations immediately preceding the outcome studies offered the opportunity not only to assess each site's capacity to carry out an outcome study, but also to identify the supported housing models that best fit the cross-site definition. The process phase provided time at the cross-site level to develop a shared understanding of the logic model guiding the study and the study interview protocols.

Finally, this chapter demonstrates how the collaborative structure in a multisite study can contribute to innovative design and analytic strategies to deal with the struggles inherent in studying dynamic and complex interventions.

Background and Description of the CMHS Housing Initiative

The CMHS Housing Initiative is a two-phase, multisite initiative designed to advance knowledge on supported housing and other housing approaches for adults with serious mental illness. Supported housing, emphasizing consumer choice, the use of regular housing stock, and individualized and flexible services and community supports, has been offered as an alternative to the traditional residential continuum, developed in response to the need for both treatment and housing for persons with serious mental illness (Carling, 1990, 1993; Hogan and Carling, 1992; Ridgeway and Zipple, 1990).

After deinstitutionalization, many persons with serious mental illness did not make a successful transition to independent living because of the lack of decent affordable housing, the lack of community-based supports, and the cyclical nature of mental illness (Dennis, Buckner, Lipton, and Levine, 1991). This situation led to the concept of the residential continuum in which community-based services are provided in a range of residential settings differentiated by the level of staffing intensity. The expectation is that consumers move through a series of progressively more independent living situations.

Preliminary research and practice have challenged the concept of the residential continuum. Many communities have not been able to create a complete continuum (Randolph and others, 1998). Moreover, the concept of the continuum may not be responsive to the varying needs of individuals (Dickey and others, 1996; Caton and Goldstein, 1984) or to their preferences or choices (Ridgeway, Simpson, Wittman, and Wheeler, 1994). Supported housing was thus developed as a strategy for allowing persons to remain in their own housing and to have services brought in as frequently and intensively as needed. The model allows individuals to choose their housing, generally dwellings that are integrated in the broader community. There is a clear and legal separation between the housing and services; no services are provided on-site. Individuals have all the rights of tenancy that are offered to any individual; specifically, they cannot be evicted or lose their housing for failure to comply with treatment. Clients may choose the services and supports they receive from those provided through an array of community-based providers.

To date, no research has rigorously compared housing approaches; the research that has examined dimensions of housing and their relationship to outcomes has been primarily descriptive. Moreover, there has been minimal attention to clearly defining what is meant by supported housing or other housing approaches.

The CMHS Housing Initiative was designed explicitly to fill this void in the knowledge base. The major policy question addressed by the initiative is whether a supported housing approach is more effective than other housing approaches in helping persons with serious mental illness achieve residential stability and improve their level of functioning, satisfaction, quality of life, and empowerment. A specific model of housing was delineated by CMHS in its 1997 Guidance for Applicants (GFA), "Cooperative Agreements to Evaluate Housing Approaches for Persons with Serious Mental Illnesses," outlining the features that defined its specific model of supported housing.

Ten sites and a coordinating center were funded in Phase I of the initiative, working collaboratively with CMHS through a steering committee.

The Housing Initiative also has the participation of a consumer advisory panel, composed of one consumer from each site.

In Phase I, each site conducted a process evaluation to demonstrate capacity to conduct a Phase II outcome evaluation and to guide the study design. In the process evaluations, sites had the opportunity to assess the proposed supported housing programs for their fit to the CMHS model and to assess the proposed comparison housing for their similarities to and differences from supported housing. The process evaluation also provided the opportunity for sites to study the target population and how adequate sample sizes could be achieved, as well as to assess the overall feasibility of mounting a rigorous outcome study following cross-site procedures.

Through a competitive process, six sites were selected for Phase II. Each site is conducting a quasi-experiment assessing supported housing and one or more comparison housing approaches. Most of the design and analytic challenges in the study stem from the difficulties that are inherent in studying housing. All housing approaches eligible to be included in the study were to have existed in the community for two years or more. Although this requirement ensured that the housing programs were up and running in the communities, it also meant that sites had to find models in their communities that met this requirement; there was little, if any, flexibility for the study teams to modify or tweak the interventions to meet study needs. Moreover, because the study population was limited to new entrants into the housing, regular turnover was needed in the housing. With tightening housing markets, turnover and vacancies can be at a premium, increasing enrollment difficulties.

Handling Challenges Faced in the Housing Initiative

The major challenges that the housing initiative faced were study design, assessment of fidelity across sites, and maintenance of effective collaboration.

Designing Studies with a Phased Approach. One of the challenges that sites confronted was identifying existing supported housing that met the study fidelity criteria. To apply for the initial GFA, the investigators in each site needed to identify one or more supported housing programs that met the criteria stated in the GFA: the consumer either owns the housing or has a lease in his or her own name; the service agency is not the housing agency; the housing is integrated into the community; services are voluntary; the consumer has a choice in the housing and in the services; services are community based; services are available for twenty-four hours; and there are no on-site services staff in the housing.

As the criteria began to be operationalized during Phase I, it was apparent that in several sites, the supported housing identified differed from the ideal supported housing model on one or more dimensions. Because the investigators rarely had the authority to change the interventions, they were often put in the position of looking for other housing or trying to increase the flexibility of the fidelity criteria to include greater variations of the supported housing approach.

One of the most difficult criteria for supported housing programs to meet in at least two of the sites was affordability, ultimately defined as housing costs (for example, rent) that are 40 percent or less of a person's adjusted income. The lack of housing subsidies in these sites, both southern cities, made it impossible to find housing that could meet the criterion. Consequently, one study withdrew after Phase I, and another was not funded for Phase II.

Although it was difficult to lose sites from Phase I to II, the process of having sites rigorously assess the feasibility of their designs—in particular, whether intervention programs could be identified to meet the criteria—helped to maintain greater integrity in the cross-site study. In addition, it provided all projects an opportunity to find housing programs that more clearly matched the study criteria, even if it meant expanding the geographical area of the study. The phased approach also helped sites to fine-tune their designs and conduct pipeline studies that would give them an idea of how many new entrants they could expect in any housing program. These studies led sites to include more housing programs than originally planned to ensure a sufficient sample size.

Strengthening Analyses Using Fidelity Data. The steering committee worked to develop a fidelity framework, based on the GFA, that incorporated the elements considered critical to the supported housing model, as well as others that were more useful in describing the comparison models. It defined each of these major components or dimensions of the housing, provided measurement indicators for each dimension, and described the measurement outcomes necessary to have a fidelity fit (that is, how closely the ideal model was approximated) on each dimension (see Table 5.1). Each indicator was operationalized at a conceptual level using a five-point scale, with a rating of 5 generally being closest to the ideal model of supported housing and 1 being furthest away.

In Phase II, a triangulated data collection methodology was adopted to assess the fidelity of supported housing and the characteristics of comparison housing. Instruments were developed to collect data from program management, staff, and resident perspectives. Interviews were conducted with a program manager and a key staff informant in each housing program in the study. Resident data were collected from study participants as part of the twelve-month follow-up interview (or in a separate exit interview if people moved out of study housing before the twelve-month interview).

Because some of the housing programs had only one study participant, it was decided that a housing program's fidelity score would be determined with program management and staff data only. Resident fidelity data would be used in outcome analyses, however.

To ensure consistency across the sites, the coordinating center developed fidelity instruments with input from the steering committee. Site-specific

Table 5.1. Housing Fidelity Dimensions and Indicators for the CMHS Housing Initiative

Dimensions	Indicators
Housing choice	Exploration of preferences Choice of units Choice of living arrangement
Housing and services separation	Legal separation Functional separation Functional separation-off-site
Integration	
Rights of tenure	Full rights of tenancy Independence Permanence in housing
Service choice	
Service individualization	Needs and preferences Agency flexibility
Community-based services	Array available Array accessible Crisis available Bundling

nuances in some of the terms used, such as *case manager* or *housing program staff,* required flexibility in defining what was meant by these terms at the individual sites to ensure uniformity and quality of data collected across the sites. The coordinating center received all completed interviews and implemented procedures for clarifying items with sites and for cleaning, coding, and data entry and analysis.

The fidelity data have strengthened the multisite evaluation in a number of ways. First, they tested the supported housing programs against an ideal, determining the extent of fidelity fit. The assessment of supported housing fidelity was initially conceived as an important feature for the Phase I study only, to ensure that only supported housing programs that met a common set of criteria were included in the multisite study. It was discovered that, in reality, there was a continuum of supported housing rather than a fit to an ideal model (see Figure 5.1).

In addition, the fidelity assessment characterized the comparison housing programs and how they compared and contrasted with supported housing (see Figure 5.1). Although the supported housing condition was well defined in the GFA, the comparison housing condition was much less prescribed, in part because of the lack of comparable attention in the field to defining the dimensions and principles of the various residential approaches. The GFA stipulated that the comparison condition could include group homes, supervised apartments, and supportive communities. What became apparent, however, is that there was very little consistency in the use of

Figure 5.1. Linear Distance from Ideal Supported Housing by
Housing Type

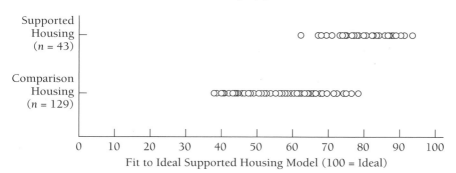

these labels across jurisdictions and even by providers in characterizing the nature of the housing. Moreover, because principles of supported housing have been widely touted, a number of the comparison housing approaches apparently have been shaped to include some of these principles and features.

Finally, the dimensional approach to measuring the housing permits an examination of the role of key housing ingredients in predicting resident outcomes. Knowing what specific features (such as having rights of tenure and having housing choice) relate to outcomes could guide the work of practitioners in refining existing housing programs to maximize their effects.

Challenges and Opportunities of Collaboration. The multisite structure set up by CMHS for this initiative, much like the others described in this volume, is a highly collaborative one in which all key cross-site decisions are made by a steering committee composed of the sites, the coordinating center, a consumer panel, and the federal government. This structure can be unwieldy and inefficient; much processing of information is needed to ensure that all individuals share the same operating assumptions and have the same base of cross-site knowledge to make decisions. In addition, balancing the need for uniformity with the variability among sites often can lead to implementing procedures that fit the lowest common denominator or the most inflexible condition.

For example, in the Housing Initiative, although collecting baseline information from residents prior to their entering housing would have been ideal, it was possible in only half of the sites. Because the steering committee thought that this variation would be detrimental to the cross-site study, all sites were required to collect baseline data after residents entered the housing, thus having all sites follow the least desirable but most uniform data collection procedure.

The collaborative structure can also strengthen the scientific quality of the study and its potential for producing relevant findings. Several examples from the Housing Initiative illustrate the value that the multisite structure can add.

First, the cross-site study can be enhanced and augmented by the individual efforts of the sites. In the Housing Initiative, site-specific qualitative studies and collection of additional data or data from other comparison groups were used to question and assess the validity of aspects of the cross-site data collection. For example, an in-depth qualitative study of the housing in one site helped to shape some of the cross-site fidelity assessment.

Second, the steering committee mechanism allows for up-to-the-minute sharing of experience and expertise that can shape individual designs and processes and, consequently, improve study implementation. An example is the sharing of information, strategies, and expertise around study recruitment. As background, the Phase I process evaluation afforded the investigators an opportunity to conduct a pipeline study (Boruch, 1997) to determine if the numbers of mentally ill persons entering and leaving the selected housing were sufficient to conduct a sensitive test of the housing approaches. In a few sites, the results of these studies led the investigators to add housing programs to one or both of the study conditions.

Even with these pipeline studies, slower-than-expected turnover in housing during Phase II occurred, causing delays in recruiting study participants and, in some sites, smaller-than-expected and often uneven samples. Within six months of recruitment, all sites but one were below the projected goal. A meeting of the steering committee focused on understanding the problems and developing strategies to increase the sample size. Among the problems that sites faced were not learning about vacancies from providers in a timely fashion (if at all), not getting referrals from case managers, and the tightening of the housing market, leading to longer housing stays, less turnover, and fewer vacancies for the study.

Strategies shared by sites included ways for projects to be more proactive in learning about vacancies (such as having staff located at the site and sending routine fax-back memos concerning new move-ins and expected move-outs), to have set scripts for case managers to use in describing the study to prospective study participants to obtain a consent to contact, and to increase the possible vacancies through expanding the number of housing programs, providers, or geographical regions in the study.

The collaborative structure can also strengthen the analysis of the data, pooling expertise from the individual study sites and their respective organizations, as well as providing the resources for, and attracting the interest of, high-level consultants. From the outset, over half of the sites in the Housing Initiative deemed it infeasible to conduct a randomized study of housing. The impracticalities and ethical problems of withholding available housing, the speed with which some housing decisions were made, and the unwillingness of providers and others to follow a randomized placement process were all factors that led sites to implement quasi-experimental studies. In a few sites, randomized studies were initially proposed but could not be implemented. In one site where many individuals continued to live in institutions, officials in the state mental health system agreed to the process and saw it as a way to place people into the community quickly. However, staff and housing providers were not as easy to convince; putting individuals from hospitals into their own housing without first going through a continuum was viewed as inappropriate. The study ultimately ended because of the difficulties in mounting the randomization. In yet another study, randomization was in place at the outset of the study but was subsequently abandoned because of changes that managed care companies in the system were facing.

Therefore, all sites either began or ended up with a quasi-experimental approach to studying the housing. All sites proposed to use a propensity scoring approach to strengthen their studies (Rubin, 1997), a procedure that entails statistically matching the individuals between treatment and control groups on a propensity score constructed from many covariates. The challenge we have collectively faced is in developing a cross-site propensity scoring approach that is feasible and meaningful. Because this is new statistical territory, having statistical expertise from many organizations has sharpened our thinking and led to a critical, systematic approach to developing propensity scores. Experts have been contacted to review the approach and offer guidance, generally in the form of confirming what we have done and helping us to determine appropriate methods to evaluate the approach we have used.

Finally, a key element of the Housing Initiative multisite structure is an active consumer panel, composed of a representative from each of the study sites. This panel has been involved since the beginning of the initiative and has provided input into the cross-site logic model, the instrumentation, study implementation, and the analyses and results interpretation, among other study aspects. For example, the panel has been working with other steering committee members to develop a combined outcome measure from a set of subjective measures as an attempt to reduce the number of measures and to handle the multicollinearity among the measures. They have deliberated on the appropriate weighting for various scales and subscales to develop a score that would represent the relative importance of these various outcomes (for example, empowerment, housing satisfaction). By the active involvement of consumers in multisite collaboration, the Housing Initiative has the potential for producing findings that are more grounded and relevant to the lives of individuals with mental illness who are in need of housing.

In the best of circumstances, the collaborative structure offered through prospective multisite evaluations creates an invisible college (Reiss and Boruch, 1991) in which a community of researchers, practitioners, and consumers shares its knowledge and expertise for the greater good.

Lessons Learned

The CMHS Housing Initiative offers a number of lessons for designing and conducting prospective multisite evaluations. First, it has reinforced the importance of a phased approach to these complex efforts. Although the incorporation of a process evaluation in the study does not guarantee that problems will not occur in the outcome study (as seen with the overestimation of the sites' ability to recruit sufficient numbers within the allotted time frame), it does provide critical information in helping sites develop more feasible designs. In some instances, it even provides enough information to persuade a site not to conduct the study.

Second, the study has reminded us of a well-worn phrase for social psychologists, coined by Kurt Lewin, stating that there is nothing as practical as a good theory. This is true for applied research, as well as for basic research, and is at least as important for multisite studies as it is for individual studies. In multisite evaluations, program theory can be the cross-site unifier in all aspects of the study. In the Housing Initiative, the inclusion of this theory in the original GFA provided the impetus for each site to propose a similar intervention and outcome assessment plan.

Moreover, the attention given to assessing the dimensions of all housing approaches has enhanced the study's ability to understand the key ingredients of housing that may improve residents' stability, empowerment, independence, functioning, and satisfaction in housing. Being able to break down these approaches into their specific elements is consistent with Weiss's calls (1997) for understanding how programs operate and affect outcomes. Knowledge of these ingredients can inform replication efforts by providing information on how providers can modify their interventions to include or enhance these ingredients. By making key changes rather than having to adopt entire new models of intervention, it is likely that more providers would be receptive to the results and the ways they could incorporate them into their existing operations. The Housing Initiative is just beginning to try to examine these ingredients and how they relate to outcomes. One of the challenges is balancing the desire for testing a number of specific ingredients of the housing initiative with the analytic challenges of having too many terms in the model. Using structural equation models or similar techniques may help in this area, but we may still find ourselves with unwieldy models and the need to select certain ingredients for examination.

Finally, the Housing Initiative provides another example of the difficulty of designing and implementing multisite evaluations; they take more time, energy, and commitment than individual studies because of the need to communicate and work closely with many diverse parties sharing different philosophies about research, interventions, and populations. As analyses are under way, our steering committee has begun a pattern of two or three two-hour conference calls each month to review analytic results and issues. With a clear structure, leadership, lines of communication and a chain of communication command, and clarity of roles (Kraemer, 2000), multisite studies can be powerful collaborative vehicles for accelerating understanding in a field of inquiry with studies that are likely to be better designed, more carefully designed, and more carefully and widely reported in policy, practice, and research outlets.

Conclusion

In the Housing Initiative, the close working relationships of the sites, the coordinating center, the federal government, and the consumer panel have ensured that multiple perspectives and expertise have been infused into the research and have helped to counter the many challenges the study has confronted. Without this collaboration, it is unlikely that there would have been as painstaking an approach to fidelity assessment or such a shared commitment to the cross-site study in general. The development of mutual respect and trust, as well as an esprit de corps, has created a working environment that is ripe for collective ideas and action. The synergy gained by coming together has likely strengthened each of the individual efforts and strengthened the potential for the cross-site study to improve policy and programs for individuals living with serious mental illness.

References

Boruch, R. F. "Randomized Experiments for Planning and Evaluation: A Practical Guide." In L. Bickman and D. Rog (Eds.), *Applied Social Research Method Series* (Vol. 44). Thousand Oaks, Calif.: Sage, 1997.

Carling, P. J. "Major Mental Illness, Housing, and Supports: The Promise of Community Integration." *American Psychologist*, 1990, *45*, 969–975.

Carling, P. J. "Housing and Supports for Persons with Mental Illness: Emerging Approaches to Research and Practice." *Hospital and Community Psychiatry*, 1993, *44*, 439–449.

Caton, C.L.M., and Goldstein, J. "Housing Change of Chronic Schizophrenic Patients: A Consequence of the Revolving Door." *Social Science and Medicine*, 1984, *19*, 759–764.

Dennis, D., Buckner, J., Lipton, F. R., and Levine, I. S. "A Decade of Research and Services for Homeless Mentally Ill Persons: Where Do We Stand?" *American Psychologist*, 1991, *46*, 1129–1138.

Dickey, B., and others. "Use of Mental Health Services by Formerly Homeless Adults Residing in Group and Independent Housing." *Psychiatric Services*, 1996, *47*, 152–158.

Edwards, P. "Conceptual and Methodological Issues in Evaluating Emergent Programs." *Evaluation and Program Planning*, 1987, *10*, 27–34.

Hogan, M. F., and Carling, P. J. "Normal Housing: A Key Element of Supported Housing Approach for People with Psychiatric Disabilities." *Community Mental Health Journal*, 1992, *28*, 215–226.

Kraemer, H. C. "Pitfalls of Multisite Randomized Clinical Trials of Efficacy and Effectiveness." *Schizophrenia Bulletin*, 2000, *26*, 535–543.

Newman, S. "Housing and Mental Illness: A Critical Review of the Literature." Unpublished manuscript, 2001.

Randolph, F., and others. *A Survey of Selected Community Residential Programs for Persons with Prolonged Mental Illness*. Boston: Center for Psychiatric Rehabilitation, Boston University, 1998.

Reiss, A. J., and Boruch, R. "The Program Review Team Approach and Multisite Experiments: The Spouse Assault Replication Program." In R. S. Turpin and J. M. Sinacore (Eds.), *Multisite Evaluations*. New Directions for Evaluation, no. 50. San Francisco: Jossey-Bass, 1991.

Ridgeway, P., Simpson, A., Wittman, F. D., and Wheeler, G. "Home Making and Community Building: Notes on Empowerment and Place." *Journal of Mental Health Administration*, 1994, *21*, 407–418.

Ridgeway, P., and Zipple, A. M. "The Paradigm Shift in Residential Services: From the Linear Continuum to Supported Housing Approaches." *Psychological Rehabilitation Journal*, 1990, *13*(4), 11–31.

Rog, D. J. "Expanding the Boundaries of Evaluation: Strategies for Refining and Evaluating Ill-Defined Interventions." In S. L. Friedman and H. C. Haywood (Eds.), *Developmental Follow-Up: Concepts, Domains, and Methods*. Orlando, Fla.: Academic Press, 1994.

Rog, D. J., Holupka, C. S., and Brito, M. C. "The Impact of Housing on Health: Examining Supportive Housing for Individuals with Mental Illness." *Current Issues in Public Health*, 1996, *2*, 153–160.

Rubin, D. "Estimating Causal Effects from Large Data Sets Using Propensity Scores." *Annals of Internal Medicine*, 1997, *127*, 757–763.

Weiss, C. H. "Theory-Based Evaluation: Past, Present, and Future." *Progress and Future Directions in Evaluation: Perspectives on Theory, Practice, and Methods*, 1997, *76*, 41–55.

DEBRA J. ROG is a senior research associate at the Vanderbilt University Institute for Public Policy Studies, where she directs the Washington, D.C., office of the Center for Mental Health Policy.

FRANCES L. RANDOLPH is acting chief of the Homeless Programs Branch, Center for Mental Health Services, Substance Abuse and Mental Health Services Administration, U.S. Department of Health and Human Services.

6

*The Center for Substance Abuse Treatment
Methamphetamine Treatment Project, with seven sites
and more than a thousand participants, is an evaluation
of a manualized psychosocial outpatient approach for the
treatment of methamphetamine-dependent individuals.*

A Multisite Evaluation of Treatment of Methamphetamine Dependence in Adults

*Richard A. Rawson, Patricia J. Marinelli-Casey,
Alice Huber*

The spread of methamphetamine (MA) production and use throughout the western and midwestern United States during the 1990s received far less attention than the cocaine-crack epidemic of the 1980s. However, from a public health perspective, the damage to the communities and individuals as a result of these drug problems has been comparable. Many parts of the country that have been besieged by problems with MA, particularly western and midwestern cities and rural areas, were ill prepared to meet the criminal justice, medical, psychiatric, social, and treatment needs created by MA use. There was very little research information to guide policymakers on how to respond properly to this crisis. Little attention had been given to the clinical problem of MA abuse for two decades, and consequently, there were few insights that could be applied to the treatment needs of individuals who sought help in the 1990s.

The Office of National Drug Control Policy led the call to attention regarding the MA problem. As a result of these efforts, attention to the

This project and research were supported by the Center for Substance Abuse Treatment (CSAT), Substance Abuse and Mental Health Services Administration (SAMHSA), cooperative agreement no. TI11440 to M. Douglas Anglin and Richard Rawson, and by CSAT contract no. 270–01–7089 to UCLA Integrated Substance Abuse Treatment Programs; Patricia Marinelli-Casey and Richard Rawson, principal investigators. The interpretations and conclusions presented in this chapter are the views of the authors and do not necessarily represent the official policy or position of SAMHSA.

problem increased dramatically, and resources have been mobilized to address it. Consequently, substantial steps have been taken to generate a better understanding of MA abuse and dependence and how to help individuals who are seeking treatment assistance. One of the most important steps for addressing the treatment needs of MA users is the MA treatment initiative, established by the Center for Substance Abuse Treatment (CSAT).

A confluence of circumstances led CSAT to solicit applications to participate in a study of the clinical and cost-effectiveness of MA treatment. First, national and regional epidemiological data indicated that MA abuse was a significant and growing problem in the United States (Anglin and others, 1998; Substance Abuse and Mental Health Services Administration, 1999; Burke and others, 2000). Second, there was no rigorously validated, well-described approach to the outpatient treatment. Third, the Matrix Institute in Los Angeles, with support from the National Institute on Drug Abuse, adapted a manualized outpatient cocaine-dependence treatment model for treating MA users and had some preliminary supportive data (Rawson and others, 1989, 1995; Huber and others, 1997). Finally, the project was designed to be responsive to the issues raised in a report from the Institute of Medicine (Lamb and others, 1998), which encouraged a greater integration of research knowledge and clinical practice.

The Matrix Institute model consists of relapse-prevention groups, education groups, social support groups, individual counseling, and urine and breath testing delivered in a structured manner over a sixteen-week period. The treatment is a directive, nonconfrontational approach that focuses on current issues and behavior change. The model has been extensively used in southern California for more than fifteen years, and both cocaine and MA users have responded well to it (Huber and others, 1997). Although some empirical support for the model had been collected, no rigorous evaluation of the treatment approach for MA dependence had been conducted. In this context, in 1998, CSAT initiated the Methamphetamine Treatment Project (MTP), a multisite study of the efficacy and effectiveness of the Matrix model. A key focus of MTP was to have sufficient scientific rigor incorporated in the design, implementation, and evaluation of the study to allow for adequate assessment of the Matrix treatment model.

Original Project Intent and Design

The purpose of CSAT's proposed program, as described in Guidance for Applicants (GFA) no. TI 98–002, "Cooperative Agreement for Replication of Effective Treatment for Methamphetamine Dependence and Improvement of Cost-Effectiveness of Treatment," was to conduct a three-year collaborative multisite study with the following goals: (1) conduct a scientifically rigorous study of the clinical effectiveness of the Matrix model for the treatment of MA abuse; (2) compare the effectiveness of the Matrix model to other locally available outpatient treatments of MA abuse; (3) establish the cost and cost-effectiveness of the Matrix approach compared to the locally available treatments; and (4) explore the replicability of the Matrix model and problems posed in technology transfer.

The GFA proposed a comparison of the sixteen-week Matrix model, an eight-week model derived from that approach, and the treatment-as-usual approach already in use by the individual study sites. Applicants were required to describe their usual approach and document their use of the approach for at least two years prior to submitting an application. The GFA also called for a coordinating center, responsible for assisting CSAT in the integration of the multiple study sites into a coherent, cohesive multisite study group.

CSAT awarded cooperative agreements to seven study sites and a coordinating center, as shown in Table 6.1. When work on MTP began in October 1998, CSAT employed an organizational structure and an implementation process that had been successfully employed and continually refined by CSAT through its experiences with other multisite studies (Rickards and others, 1999; Hanrahan and others, 1999). The standard structure consists of CSAT, the study sites, the coordinating center, and a

Table 6.1. Methamphetamine Treatment Project: Grantees and Key Personnel

Coordinating Center	Principal Investigators	Project Director
UCLA Integrated Substance Abuse Programs, Los Angeles	M. Douglas Anglin, Richard A. Rawson, UCLA	Patricia Marinelli-Casey, UCLA

Grantee	Principal Investigator	Lead Evaluator
South Central Regional Mental Health Center, Billings, Montana	Denna Vandersloot, South Central Regional Mental Health Center	Russell H. Lord, Montana State University, Billings
New Leaf Treatment Center, Concord, California	Gantt Galloway, New Leaf Treatment Center	Janice Stalcup, New Leaf Treatment Center
Matrix Center, Costa Mesa, California	Michael McCann, Matrix Center	Vikas Gulati, Matrix Center
East Bay Community Recovery Project, Hayward, California	Joan Zweben, East Bay Community Recovery Project	Judith Cohen, East Bay Community Recovery Project
St. Francis Medical Center, Honolulu, Hawaii	Alice Dickow, St. Francis Women's Addiction Treatment Center, Honolulu	Ewa Stamper, St. Francis Women's Addiction Treatment Center, Honolulu
San Diego Association of Governments, San Diego, California	Susan Pennell, San Diego Association of Governments	Cynthia Burke, San Diego Association of Governments
County of San Mateo, Belmont, California	Yvonne Frazier, County of San Mateo, Alcohol and Drug Services	Joseph Guydish, University of California, San Francisco

steering committee. Additional elements of the structure created for MTP are a scientific advisory board, a community advisory board, and several forms of technical support provided by CSAT.

The Modified MTP Project Design

MTP brought together a group of clinicians, researchers, and CSAT project staff to create a project that would allow rigorous scientific methodology to be used to evaluate treatments for MA use in a way that responded to the realities of the community treatment settings where the users sought help. At the first project steering committee meeting in October 1998, a major focus of discussion was the consideration of the specific study design.

Design Issues. Treatment providers and scientists often consider problems differently, and their approaches to the resolution of problems can also vary. Scientists desire a pure design in a large sample, exact replication of the model at each site, and measurements conducted with exactitude and at sufficient frequency across a significant duration so that the analyses can unambiguously answer the proposed questions. Treatment providers want effective and cost-effective treatments, with the flexibility to adapt services to fit the needs and expectations of their specific client populations and to adjust criteria as defined for the project (for example, inclusion and exclusion, treatment times, and frequency). The focus for the clinicians is the provision of service to a needy population. The task of the steering committee became one of finding a balance between these two perspectives.

In its grant announcement for the project, CSAT instructed applicants to propose a study that would compare the sixteen-week Matrix model, the eight-week Matrix model, and treatment as usual in a manner that could be reasonably conducted in their treatment organization. At the first steering committee meeting, it became apparent that each of the seven organizations had somewhat different ideas about the project it was planning to conduct. For example, some sites proposed plans in which candidates self-selected treatment conditions; in other sites, there was a plan to use a random assignment of subjects to treatment conditions. In other settings, the plan was that both treatment conditions would not be equally available across all sites.

Deciding on a Randomized Clinical Trial. To facilitate a rapid decision about the nature of the design, the coordinating center principal investigators presented a proposed common protocol: a multisite, three-group (Matrix eight-week program, Matrix sixteen-week program, and treatment as usual) random assignment project with a common assessment battery, in which each of the seven organizations would commit to the enrollment of a minimum of 150 participants per site. The rationale for this design was that because there were no clearly established efficacy data to support either version of the Matrix model, it was essential to determine the fundamental issue of efficacy before moving to the evaluation of cost-effectiveness or other treatment services. An important contributing factor to the selection of this design was the unanimous recommendation of the project's scientific advisory board to pursue it. Although this randomized clinical trials design was quite different from the design proposed by some of the site principal investigators, there was rapid consensus on this critical issue.

Another substantial protocol change was the decision to reduce the number of treatment conditions from three (Matrix eight- and sixteen-week and treatment as usual) to a two-group comparison. For a variety of practical and logistical reasons, the three-group comparison was deemed excessively complex. As a result, the eight-week Matrix condition was dropped from the study, and the final design became a two-group randomized comparison (Matrix sixteen-week program versus treatment as usual).

In addition to determining the efficacy of the Matrix approaches, MTP was mandated in the GFA to address two other research themes: to measure the costs of each model and the relationship between costs and outcomes and to collect information on the challenges of conducting controlled research in community treatment settings (the research-practice agenda). The creation of a study to compare the efficacy of the Matrix sixteen-week treatment protocol with treatment as usual, while simultaneously measuring the cost-effectiveness and research-to-practice implications of the project, was not viewed as feasible by the steering committee. With the approval of CSAT, the steering committee elected to focus first on conducting a solid two-group efficacy trial and then phasing in the other two project aspects.

Study Measures, Data Collection, and Management Procedures. The steering committee solicited ideas for the study measures and the data collection process. The group wanted to maximize the scope of information obtained while minimizing the burden on participants, but common data collection was necessary in order to compare data across the sites. We first considered the maximum time that we wanted to spend on collecting baseline data and the priorities among all possible domains. We agreed that three hours would be the maximum amount of time allowed for the baseline and follow-up batteries.

The primary question regarding the efficacy of the programs led the steering committee to focus on measures of drug use during and after treatment. Urinalyses to determine the use of MA, cocaine, opiates, and benzodiazepines were completed at baseline, at each week, and at follow-ups. During the treatment period, so that MA use could be tested, urine samples were collected weekly on a semirandom (that is, nonpredictable) basis. If the participant refused to provide a sample or provided an invalid sample, the sample was considered positive for MA use for data-analytic purposes.

Another focus for assessment was the participant's functioning in other areas of life. The primary measure used for this domain was the Addiction Severity Index (ASI) (McLellan and others, 1989, 1992). ASI is a structured clinical interview that reviews seven areas of life functioning: medical status, employment status, drug and alcohol use, family history, family and social relationships, legal status, and psychiatric status. We included two standardized measures of psychological problems, the Brief Symptom Inventory (Derogatis, 1993) and the Beck Depression Inventory (Beck and Steer, 1993). To assess clients' overall physical and mental health, we used the Short-Form Health Survey (Ware, Snow, Kosinski, and Gandek, 1993). To assess the occurrence of risk behaviors for human immunodeficiency virus (HIV) and exposure to domestic violence, we used a subset of items from the Women's Interagency HIV Study (WIHS) (Barkan and others, 1998) and the Texas Christian University HIV/AIDS Risk Assessment (Simpson, 1997).

We finalized the common battery of treatment process and outcome measures within ninety days of the first steering committee meeting. Each site obtained approval for the project from a local institutional review board, and the coordinating center obtained separate approval for its role in the project. All participants provided informed consent before the collection of any data. We administered the battery of instruments at baseline, treatment discharge, and six and twelve months following randomization.

The Treatment-as-Usual Problem. CSAT originally proposed an evaluation of two models of Matrix treatment and the usual treatment at the site. The Matrix sixteen-week model is manualized, so with standardized training and close clinical monitoring across the sites, this seemed feasible. However, as Galloway and others (2000) noted, the treatments as usual are markedly heterogeneous across sites, making it scientifically inadvisable to merge data from widely varying treatment-as-usual protocols. For example, one site offered weekly individual sessions of one-hour duration for a period of twelve weeks; a second site provided group sessions over a one-year period starting with daily meetings and decreasing frequency over time. The treatments varied in format (group versus individual), duration (between four and fifty-two weeks), intensity (one hour per week versus up to ten hours per week), frequency (daily versus weekly), and focus (psychodynamic versus cognitive behavioral) and thereby eluded easy characterization. As might be expected, each treatment organization was committed to employing its approach to treatment, and so there was little interest in implementing a common standard treatment at different sites. Furthermore, variation across several key dimensions was so great that the seven approaches could not be distilled into a single standard platform.

The central question that this issue brought into focus was the discrepancy between the desire of CSAT and the researchers to conduct a multisite randomized clinical trial that would be uniformly conducted across all sites and the desire of practitioners to compare a new treatment approach with the standard treatment that they delivered in their clinics. These two goals were mutually exclusive. The compromise that we reached was in the direction of accommodating the real-world consideration of the different treatments as usual and comparing the standardized Matrix sixteen-week protocol to seven different treatments as usual. Rather than a single multisite trial with two identical treatment conditions, the design became a seven-site, multiple replication model, in which each site compares the Matrix sixteen-week protocol and its usual treatment. Essentially, the project became seven parallel studies with common measures.

The use of multiple treatments as usual will allow the project to produce evidence that speaks to the relative efficacy of the manualized approach to seven different forms of community treatment. If each site successfully collects an adequate sample size to give the necessary statistical power (estimated to be 150 per site), the project will deliver seven studies in one, with a tremendous breadth of application. This is one example of where the need to compromise the traditional purity of clinical trials research design to accommodate real-world considerations may result in a more valuable study for the field.

Sample Size and Recruitment Issues. The study design called for the recruitment of 150 MA-dependent participants at each site. This sample size allows for a comparison of main effects, with an expected rate of 80 percent of participants completing follow-up. At the beginning of the study, almost all of the applicant organizations were confident, on the basis of local epidemiology and referral data, that they would have a more than adequate number of treatment-seeking MA users once the study started. This optimism was tempered by the experience of researchers who recounted many examples of inadequate research participation in spite of an overwhelming perception that there were many eligible study applicants in a particular project catchment area. The research team adamantly pushed for many and varied strategies to ensure necessary project recruitment. These efforts have been fruitful in that the projected samples were successfully achieved at most sites.

Data Analysis Challenges. The design of MTP poses several analytical challenges. The broadest and most critical among them is the conceptual design of the statistical comparison used to analyze the primary outcome. In most multisite clinical trial designs, both (or all) treatment conditions are implemented at each site. Such a design can be easily analyzed with an analysis of variance (ANOVA) approach, pooling all data together from all of the sites and analyzing the difference between the treatment arms while statistically controlling for site in order to account for suspected, known, or unknown site factors that might affect outcomes.

MTP differs from this traditional multisite clinical trial design. All sites in MTP are implementing the Matrix treatment model as one arm of the study. The treatment delivered to the comparison group at each site, however, is treatment as usual. Although it would be possible to use the standard site-controlled ANOVA approach, comparing Matrix to treatment as usual, it is not clear that this approach would yield a valid result. The treatment-as-usual approaches used at the sites vary so widely that the only valid analysis might require separate comparisons between Matrix and treat-ment as usual at each site. Modeling or meta-analysis could then be used to further understanding of the messages in the data.

Shifting from one large multisite analysis to comparisons among the conditions within each site has potentially serious disadvantages. One is the potential reduction in the statistical power of the study. The sample size of the study was set to provide sufficient power for an overall multisite analysis. It might be the case that analyzing within sites, with resultant smaller sample sizes in each comparison, may provide insufficient power to detect an effect, even if one exists. Another potential disadvantage is that results from these within-site comparisons will still need to be aggregated in some way after the fact in order to answer the primary questions of the project. It is not clear how the primary study question will be answered if there is a diversity of outcomes in the seven comparisons. Although it might indeed be the fact that site-specific factors directly affected the result, this important piece of information can be definitively statistically demonstrated only through multisite analyses. Discussions are under way concerning which of the imperfect solutions offers the fewest disadvantages.

Lessons of Implementation

Five major lessons were learned in the implementation of MTP.

Trust. Trust among researchers (coordinating center and site evalua-tors), among clinicians (coordinating center clinical directors and site cli-nicians), and between researchers and clinicians must be earned over time and is not easily established. The fact that there would be a period of time required to build trust between the researchers and the clinicians was no surprise. We anticipated that there would be many issues to negotiate and many challenges to producing a smooth working relationship between these two groups. An unexpected surprise was that there was an equivalent, if not greater, effort required to build trust between the coordinating cen-ter and some of the site evaluators and site clinical leadership.

At the core of the difficulty in some of these relationships was the aggressive timetable of the project, imposed by CSAT, and the resultant forceful stance taken by the coordinating center leadership. This caused some of the site researchers to appear to feel pressured into a project design with specific components that did not receive adequate discussion and debate. Over the course of the first year, a great deal of progress was made in building trust among project participants. Among the key ingredients to building the trust was a genuine desire on the part of all parties to make the project succeed. A paramount consideration was the near-universal desire to help improve the care available for the treatment of MA use disorders. This overriding concern for the well-being of the project participants was instrumental in the creation of a project esprit de corps.

Mutual Respect. Although every member of the project staff readily acknowledged the need for collaboration based on respect for research and clinical perspectives, conveying that attitude was often difficult. There are a number of excellent examples in an Institute of Medicine report (Lamb, Greenlick, and McCarty, 1998) of how wary community treatment providers are of working with researchers. Common adjectives that community program staff used to describe their experiences with researchers include *arrogant, condescending, disinterested in clients, rigid, disrespectful, elitist, irrelevant,* and *disrespectful of clinical staff.* Researchers have their own misgivings about clinicians. Researcher comments commonly heard are that clinicians are disorganized, ideological, unstructured, nonsystematic, and unaccountable for the services they provide. These attitudes and beliefs need to be acknowledged, challenged, discussed, and resolved as part of the process of creating a common ground of cooperation between researchers and clinicians.

The coordinating center leadership comprises a combination of clinicians, researchers, and clinician-researchers with extensive experience in conducting research trials in community-based settings. This team was sensitized to the delicacy needed in bringing researchers and clinicians together to work on projects. In the project planning activities, extensive preparations were made by the coordinating center to avoid offending community treatment program staff by maintaining a respectful stance toward working within their settings. Even with this extensive experience and the preparations, there were some rough points in the initial interactions between the coordinating center and the community treatment organizations (Zweben and others, 2000).

Cost and Complexity. Conducting research in community-based treatment settings results in additional and more complex work that can be considerably more expensive than other approaches. Community organization staff members generally have heavy workloads, and a research project within the clinic is not their only priority. Researchers may see the benefits of the outcomes of research projects but may fail to appreciate the negative implications associated with the introduction of new people, more meetings, and perhaps a different sort of client.

The logistical, technical, and communication needs of a multisite project are enormous. Time-consuming operational problems between the coordinating center and the community sites contributed substantially to major morale problems and research-clinician conflict. It is important to simplify and standardize communications with e-mail, e-mail lists, faxes, and telephone calls. Data collection and transmission systems should be operationalized only after any technical problems have been worked out. Every effort should be made to limit and facilitate the tasks required by the community organizations. The coordinating center should absorb any tasks or costs that can be handled at that level to ease the burden placed on the community agencies.

Multiple chains of command can result in undermining of authority, confusion, or resentment. A site director, research investigator, clinical supervisor, and research coordinator each have authority that sometimes overlaps for individual employees. It is important that supervisors not overstep their realms of authority. It is often necessary to redirect employees to the most appropriate supervisor, to communicate with other supervisors, and to inform the site director of staffing, scheduling, and other matters affecting the day-to-day operation of the clinic.

Adaptation. Researchers may need to be more flexible and operate more democratically than they are accustomed to. Modifications in study design may be required by community organizations to fit their clinical situations better. Some of these clinically recommended changes may make the protocol more complicated, but they may also make the project more valuable.

There are an extraordinary number of judgment calls in conducting any clinical research project. To the extent possible, decisions should be made within the context of the steering committee or in conference calls. Answering questions and making decisions in this context increase the understanding of the rationale for a decision, improve acceptance of the new outcome, and increase procedural standardization across sites. The number of questions that can be brought into this context is related to the degree to which a supportive, interactive relationship can be established and maintained.

Training on Interpersonal Issues. Research and clinical staff members may have conflicts regarding relationships with mutual patients-subjects. The interpersonal relationship that develops between study participants and the research staff can be difficult for clinical staff. As expected, clients share confidential information with research staff in a one-to-one relationship. Some clinical staff may be threatened by this relationship, and this issue should be openly discussed between the research and clinical staff at the site on an ongoing basis.

At times, research assistants may drift into a quasi-counselor role with research subjects. They may feel flattered by comparisons to the counselor in which they are supposedly preferred. Sometimes they can unknowingly contribute to an undermining of the counselor's effectiveness and interfere with the client's recovery. The potential negative effects of this predictable situation can be minimized by adequate training and supervision of research staff.

Additional Study Components

The steering committee focused first on conducting the randomized clinical trial, delaying implementation of the cost-effectiveness and research-practice interface components of the project. Once the primary study was initiated, the group initiated the procedures to accomplish these other features.

The Cost-Effectiveness Element. Measures were needed to determine the efficacy and cost-effectiveness of the programs. Several measures were already integrated in the primary study to assess treatment service delivery. The first, the Treatment Services Review (McLellan and others, 1989), is a standardized instrument in which the participant is asked what services were received in the preceding week (within the program and external to the program), categorized according to the seven problem areas on the ASI. As a second measure, the clinical chart is reviewed to determine the clinical services delivered, as indicated in the clinical notes. The treatment tracking forms were modified at each site to match the types of services offered.

In addition to the delineation of services provided and received, we needed information about costs (from both the program and client perspective) and perceived benefits to complete the analyses. We asked participants about their perception of the treatment received, using the Client Satisfaction Questionnaire and the Services Evaluation Questionnaire (Attkisson and Greenfield, 1994), and about their estimation of the time and money spent to attend the program, using the Drug Abuse Treatment Cost Analysis Program–Client Version (French, 2001). The implementation of these specific cost-effectiveness components occurred in year 2 of the project. The outcomes of the full cost-benefit analyses are still pending.

Qualitative Evaluation of Research-Practice Interface. CSAT and the steering committee thought that the project presented an excellent opportunity to collect important science-into-practice data by answering questions such as the following:

As scientific inquiry becomes an integral component of counseling intervention, how do counselors and administrators react to new challenges created by implementing scientific inquiry in the midst of therapy?

How do clinicians respond when working in a context of ongoing scientific inquiry that requires careful monitoring of consistent protocols across multiple sites and counselors?

How does the everyday life of a provider agency change when the agency is involved in the scientific testing of a preferred treatment with a different treatment?

Because traditional scientific methodology is not well suited for assessing these issues, the steering committee decided to embed a qualitative component within MTP.

This qualitative component involves interviews with a carefully chosen small sample at each site (for example, project directors and evaluators, agency administrators) to obtain a depiction of the practical, everyday impacts of the project. The field notes gathered in these open-ended interviews will provide a picture of MTP that is different from and not addressed by standardized questionnaires. These interviews were conducted by an independent qualitative researcher in years 2 and 3.

The Added Value of MTP

The application of the Matrix model to this trial is one of the first systematic attempts to take a clinical protocol developed through the National Institute on Drug Abuse into a CSAT-funded effectiveness trial. The study design that was chosen to test the model has the promise of producing systematic data on the implementation of the Matrix approach in multiple settings, with diverse cultural and ethnic groups and with voluntary and mandated treatment populations. In addition to the information on the Matrix approach, the project provides important preliminary evaluation information on seven other clinical approaches for the treatment of MA abuse and dependence. The experiences based on this multisite project will also provide a model for transferring research-based treatments into community settings.

Although the choice of the multisite replication design, with different treatment-as-usual conditions, creates significant analysis challenges, it does allow for multiple individual site and model comparisons. Given the early stage in the development of empirically supported treatments for MA dependence, the information from this multiple comparison design may have benefits unavailable in more traditional designs.

The study that is being conducted in this project employs a level of training, monitoring, data collection, and protocol adherence that has not heretofore been implemented in community treatment settings. Key researchers, clinicians, and policymakers continue to debate how to eliminate the research-practice gap, but there has been little visible progress. In contrast, this is one of the first systematic attempts to identify the minefields and recognize where areas of cooperation exist.

The qualitative evaluation and the cost-effectiveness components are two other unique aspects of the project. The information to be collected by these aspects of the project will further inform the discussion about how those conducting treatment feel about research. This element of the project has the promise of bringing the actual experience of clinicians involved in a research project into what has been almost exclusively a debate fueled by conjecture and rhetoric. The cost-effectiveness component of the project is probably the most ambitious and most difficult to accomplish. However, the information regarding the cost of providing evidence-based treatments in real-world settings will augment the existing data considerably. Furthermore, it will enhance what is known about how to measure this dimension of project effectiveness.

As of this writing, MTP continues to treat clients and collect data. A number of data-analytic strategies have been discussed, and a final decision is still pending. From an evaluation perspective, the best-case scenario is for the Matrix model either to produce superior treatment outcomes at all seven sites or to produce worse ones—a result that would definitively establish the value of the Matrix model for the field. The worst-case scenario would be for the Matrix model to produce clinically superior results in some sites, worse results in others, and equivalent results in the remainder, with no interpretable pattern. MTP is well positioned to take advantage of the best scenario and an intermediate possibility: that the Matrix model is at least as good as treatment as usual at all seven sites. Either of these outcomes would allow MTP to present the field with a documented treatment approach that is at least as effective as standard practice. The economic evaluation component of MTP would then enable a determination of the relative costs of treatments with equivalent or differential effectiveness. Furthermore, MTP is in part a multisite evaluation of the standardized Matrix model. Because of the wide variation in populations across sites, in gender, ethnicity, and route of administration most notably, MTP offers the opportunity to examine the effectiveness of the Matrix approach with different populations. Thus, although we still must resolve how best to analyze these data given the treatment-as-usual problem, MTP as a prospective multisite trial has the potential to offer far more than a set of stand-alone, independent studies.

The activities surrounding the project have already promoted better knowledge dissemination about MA. Along with the training that has been provided to the fifty project staff in seven locations, the project has served to prompt large-scale community training events on MA in Portland, Oregon; Honolulu, Hawaii; Billings, Montana; San Mateo County, California; and the District of Columbia. Presentations on the project have been given at a number of national conferences, and others will be forthcoming when the research data are complete. A special issue of the *Journal of Psychoactive Drugs* was published in 2000 describing in detail many of the design and early implementation issues (Anglin and Rawson, 2000).

The successes or failures of MTP will be a result of a collaborative-cooperative effort. Because of the way the program announcement was written and responded to by applicants, each of the site groups came to the project with its own ideas of what the project was about and what it wanted to do. It is safe to say that no grantee was able to proceed with the project that it had proposed. However, with assistance from the CSAT program staff, the project's steering committee was able to make many difficult decisions very rapidly. The scientific advisory board and the community advisory board played key roles in clarifying aspects of the project design and priorities. The cooperation of the site principal investigators, the site researchers, and the site clinical staff has been near universal. We wait with anticipation the outcomes of the trial, we celebrate the products and the focus that have developed to date, and we look forward to other projects that present such unique opportunities to continue the important work of blending research and practice.

References

Anglin, M. D., and others. *NEDTAC Regional Report: Epidemiology and Treatment of Methamphetamine Abuse in California*. Rockville, Md.: Center for Substance Abuse Treatment, 1998.

Anglin, M. D., and Rawson, R. A. "Editors' Introduction: The CSAT Methamphetamine

Treatment Project: Moving Research into the 'Real World.'" *Journal of Psychoactive Drugs,* 2000, *32,* 135–136.

Attkisson, C. C., and Greenfield, T. K. "The Client Satisfaction Questionnaire–8 and the Service Satisfaction Questionnaire–30." In M. E. Maurish (Ed.), *The Use of Psychological Testing for Treatment Planning and Outcome Assessment.* Mahwah, N.J.: Erlbaum, 1994.

Barkan, S. E., and others. *The Women's Interagency Study (WIHC)—1. Design, Methods, Sample.* Bethesda, Md.: WISH Collaborative Study Group, Office of AIDS Research, 1998.

Beck, A. T., and Steer, R. A. *Beck Depression Inventory Manual.* New York: Harcourt Brace, 1993.

Burke, C., and others. "History of the Methamphetamine Problem." *Journal of Psychoactive Drugs,* 2000, *32,* 137–141.

Derogatis, L. R. *Brief Symptom Inventory: Administration, Scoring, and Procedures Manual.* Minneapolis, Minn.: National Computer Systems, 1993.

French, M. T. *Drug Treatment Cost Analysis Program (DATCAP): Program Version.* (7th ed.) Coral Gables, Fla.: University of Miami, 2001.

Galloway, G. P., and others. "Treatment-as-Usual in the Methamphetamine Treatment Project." *Journal of Psychoactive Drugs,* 2000, *32,* 165–176.

Hanrahan, P., and others. "Cooperative Agreements for CMHS/CSAT Collaborative Program to Prevent Homelessness: Conclusion." *Alcoholism Treatment Quarterly,* 1999, *17,* 183–203.

Huber, A., and others. "Integrating Treatments for Methamphetamine Abuse: A Psychosocial Perspective." *Journal of Addictive Diseases,* 1997, *16*(4), 41–50.

Lamb, S., Greenlick, M. R., and McCarty, D. (Eds.). *Bridging the Gap Between Practice and Research.* Washington, D.C.: Institute of Medicine, 1998.

McLellan, A. T., and others. *Administration Manual for the Treatment Services Review.* Philadelphia: Veterans Affairs Medical Center, 1989.

McLellan, A. T., and others. "The Fifth Edition of the Addiction Severity Index." *Journal of Substance Abuse Treatment,* 1992, *9,* 199–213.

Rawson, R. A., and others. *The Neurobehavioral Treatment Manual.* Beverly Hills, Calif.: Matrix, 1989.

Rawson, R. A., and others. "An Intensive Outpatient Approach for Cocaine Abuse Treatment: The Matrix Model." *Journal of Substance Abuse Treatment,* 1995, *12,* 117–217.

Rickards, L. D., and others. "Cooperative Agreements for CMHS/CSAT Collaborative Program to Prevent Homelessness: An Overview." *Alcoholism Treatment Quarterly,* 1999, *17,* 1–15.

Simpson, D. D. "Measurement of HIV Risk Behavior." Paper presented at the National Institute on Drug Abuse Workshop, Gaithersburg, Md., Sept. 11–12, 1997.

Substance Abuse and Mental Health Services Administration. *Treatment for Stimulant Use Disorders.* Rockville, Md.: Center for Substance Abuse Treatment, 1999.

Ware, J. E., Snow, K. K., Kosinski, M., and Gandek, B. *SF-36 Health Survey Manual and Interpretation Guide.* Boston: Health Institute, New England Medical Center, 1993.

Zweben, J. E., and others. "Conducting Trials in Community Settings: The Provider Perspective." *Journal of Psychoactive Drugs,* 2000, *32,* 193–200.

RICHARD A. RAWSON *is the associate director of the University of California at Los Angeles (UCLA) Integrated Substance Abuse Programs, a program in the UCLA Department of Psychiatry and Biobehavioral Sciences, UCLA School of Medicine.*

PATRICIA J. MARINELLI-CASEY *is an assistant research psychologist at the UCLA Integrated Substance Abuse Programs.*

ALICE HUBER *is a senior research scientist with Friends Research Institute, Seattle, Washington.*

Publicly funded multisite evaluations should help bring safe, effective interventions to the mental health and substance abuse treatment fields. Two principles, science-based practice and stakeholder participation, drive multisite evaluations of behavioral interventions. We examine the roles of these principles in the five programs described in this volume and draw lessons for future studies.

Lessons Learned About Science and Participation from Multisite Evaluations

H. Stephen Leff, Virginia Mulkern

The preceding chapters present a range of multiple site evaluations and the problems encountered in their execution. Many offer creative and at least partially effective solutions to these problems. In this final chapter, we discuss our observations on these problems and potential solutions within the context of two underlying principles at work in multisite evaluations (MSEs), which are often in conflict when seeking potential remedies.

Before doing so, however, it is important to recognize that publicly funded MSEs have the purpose of bringing interventions that are proven safe and effective to the public. The problems described in the preceding chapters stem from an evolving understanding of the implications of this purpose. As this understanding evolved, it became clear that not all features of MSE designs were optimal with respect to this purpose. To the extent that investigator-initiated, single-site studies have the same purpose, they must address the same implications.

The authors thank the editors for their helpful comments. This chapter was also informed by ongoing discussions on this topic with Michael English, Neal Brown, Crystal Blyler, and Betsy McDonald, Division of Knowledge Development and Systems Change, Center for Mental Health Services (CMHS), and Mady Chalk and Fran Cotter, Center for Substance Abuse Treatment. Work on the chapter was supported in part by grant no. 6 UR1 SM53128–0202 from CMHS, Substance Abuse and Mental Health Services Administration (SAMHSA). The interpretations and conclusions contained in this chapter are the views of the authors and do not necessarily represent the position of SAMHSA.

The underlying principles that shaped these MSEs of publicly funded mental health and substance abuse services are that services should be science based and that MSEs should have broad participation by stakeholders. The concept of science-based practice is that to bring safe, effective interventions to the public, MSEs should contribute to an orderly, phased process of scientific investigation. This concept is also referred to as promoting science-based practices. It is currently driving both MSEs, particularly those sponsored by government organizations and foundations (Chapter One, this volume), and services planning and delivery.

The participatory principle is the idea that MSEs should reflect the interests and values of the various stakeholder groups in public systems, including public officials, evaluators, consumers, advocates, and family members. This idea is expressed in the concept of learning communities, described by Straw and Herrell in Chapter One. In part, this principle reflects the value that persons should participate in the institutions that affect their personal and working lives. However, it also reflects the sociological reality that evidence of effectiveness alone is rarely enough to ensure adoption of interventions. Much also depends on such social factors as political and intellectual alliances, friendships, and institutional loyalties (Bell, 1998; Godfried, 1999). Finally, it reflects the reality that when scientists, policymakers, or payers alone bring interventions to the public, providers, consumers, and members of ethnic, racial, and cultural groups become suspicious and can even reject the results of multisite and other evaluations (Godfried, 1999; Bernal and Scharro-del-Rio, 2001; Anthony, 2001).

Each of the two principles plays an important role in the development and evaluation of substance abuse and mental health interventions. However, the implications of each of these principles, taken separately and in combination, have yet to be fully articulated and translated into guidelines for planning and implementing MSEs. As the chapters in this volume illustrate, MSEs vary tremendously (see Chapters One and Four). The challenges that the evaluators have encountered reflect and illustrate the fact that these two principles and their interrelationship have yet to be fully operationalized. In this chapter, we describe each of the principles more fully, discuss the challenges that each presents using examples from this volume, and suggest next steps to improve the process of bringing proven behavioral interventions to the public.

The Science-Based Principle

The science-based principle holds that an intervention should be brought to the public through a phased process in which the intervention is (1) developed and demonstrated to be feasible, safe, and potentially effective; (2) rigorously tested against a placebo or placebo-like intervention that lacks the specific ingredients of the intervention in order to test for effectiveness; (3) compared to other effective interventions to test for equivalence or superiority; and (4) monitored in routine use for adverse events or indications of broader applicability. This approach underlies the U.S. Food and Drug Administration's approval process for new drugs and medical devices (Leff and others, 2002), as well as the more generic phases of research model described in Chapter One of this volume.

There are good reasons for advocating this structured approach to testing substance abuse and mental health interventions. First, violating this progression means that there are aspects of an intervention's safety and effectiveness that remain to be proven. Second, if all interventions must follow the progression, then intervention developers know what is expected of them and can expect competing interventions to face the same hurdles, which establishes a level playing field for competing interventions. Third, evidence about the safety and effectiveness that is produced through this type of systematic process provides a rational basis for selecting among available alternatives.

Applying the science-based principle to behavioral health interventions is more difficult than applying it to drugs and medical devices. In a number of areas, there is a lack of consensus as to exactly how to apply the science-based principle to investigations of behavioral health interventions (whether single site or multisite). Challenges related to the failure to reach consensus on how scientific methods should be applied to MSEs are discussed below.

Matching Designs to the Developmental Stage of an Intervention. The science-based principle suggests that the appropriateness of bringing an intervention to the public should be assessed through a phased series of trials. However, the idea of a phased process for evaluating behavioral interventions has not been formally established, and there is no organization with a mandate to guide the process of scientific development for behavioral interventions.[1] Therefore, MSEs tend to address a range of questions related to different intervention types and differing target populations in no particular order. As a result, some MSEs have found themselves testing interventions that had not yet been fully developed or comparing interventions when the question at issue was whether any of the interventions under study were efficacious or effective (see Chapters Three through Five, this volume).

The design of MSEs should take into account the developmental stage of the intervention. The Center for Mental Health Services Housing Initiative for persons with serious mental illness, described by Rog and Randolph in Chapter Five, illustrates the value of assessing which phases of development have been satisfied when planning an MSE. This MSE was initially implemented to address the question of whether supported housing is more effective with respect to residential stability and other outcomes than alternative housing approaches. However, it was initiated at a time when there had been minimal attention to defining clearly what was meant by supported housing or by other approaches combining housing and services and prior to any consensus that there was evidence showing that supported housing was more effective than housing without a specific connection to services. For this reason, the MSE was planned to begin with an intervention development phase. In this phase, the concept of supported housing was jointly developed by participants, as were related evaluation tools, such as fidelity measures. Once these tasks were completed, sites had to compete to go on to the intervention comparison phase.

Identifying Appropriate Program Contrasts. The strength of MSEs can best be leveraged when they are used to investigate the differential effects of clearly defined interventions and equally well-defined alternatives that are appropriate to an intervention's phase of development and provide clear contrasts with policy relevance. The MSEs described in Chapters Three, Five, and Six illustrate the lack of consensus about how to define appropriate and persuasive controls.

Employment Intervention Demonstration Program (EIDP) sites used a mixture of no service, services as usual, and alternative employment interventions as controls. Each of these comparisons presents problems. A no-services condition, like a waiting list control, does not control for expectancy effects. A services-as-usual condition can be problematic in several ways. If services are poorly implemented, services as usual may have harmful effects. And while a services-as-usual condition may control for expectancy effects, it may also contain specific ingredients of the index intervention. The use of alternative interventions as controls can also cause conceptual ambiguity if these interventions have not themselves been demonstrated as effective. Because there was no agreed-on standard defining the types of control groups that would yield unambiguous results, the EIDP mixed studies to test interventions with studies to compare alternative interventions, thus complicating the analysis and interpretability of findings.

Although it is unclear that the efficacy or effectiveness of supported housing has been tested (Newman, 2001), the supported housing MSE compared supported housing to other types of housing programs (Chapter Five, this volume). There was no requirement that these other types of housing have demonstrated efficacy or effectiveness, which would have qualified them as appropriate controls for testing the efficacy or effectiveness of supported housing. Furthermore, there was no requirement that the control housing types have certain nonspecific characteristics and lack other ones specific to supported housing, leaving it unclear as to how the control interventions differed from the index intervention. In response to this situation, the supported housing MSE developed procedures to identify critical ingredients of all interventions. This approach, while clearly in the right direction, leaves open the question of an appropriate placebo-like control group for testing the efficacy or effectiveness of supported housing or any other type. It is beyond the scope of this chapter to decide what constitutes adequate placebo-like controls for the various behavioral interventions. However, in some cases, like supported housing, this difficult problem remains to be solved.

Sites in the Marijuana Treatment Project, described by Babor and others in Chapter Two, used a waiting list control. Waiting lists are problematic proxies for placebo controls, since they do not contain nonspecific ingredients. Furthermore, persons on waiting lists may alter their behavior in anticipation of receiving treatment. The study by Rawson and others (Chapter Six) employed services-as-usual comparison groups, which ultimately resulted in questions about the meaning of the comparisons with the index intervention.

The types of program contrasts used in the MSEs described in this volume illustrate the complexity of designing behavioral evaluations that will yield unambiguous results. The issue of appropriate comparisons is not limited to MSEs. This issue simply becomes more pressing, given the considerable resources required to conduct MSEs. Agreement on some rules of thumb concerning appropriate comparisons might provide some clarity. Tests to prove the efficacy and effectiveness of interventions should give considerable thought to whether placebo-like comparison groups can be designed. Such comparison groups yield results that are much less ambiguous than other types of controls, such as waiting list controls and services as usual. If other services must be used as controls, the difference between the index intervention and the control should be understood and measured at all sites. If a comparison intervention that has been tested in comparison to a placebo-like control exists, it should be used. In any case, MSE designs that include comparison groups should require sites to employ groups that allow for meaningful cross-site comparisons.

Designing Sampling Strategies. Randomization has received more attention than have issues related to the appropriateness of control or comparison groups, despite the fact that the issue of appropriate comparisons is conceptually more difficult to address than randomization and is a logically prior question to resolve, since randomization to comparison groups that cannot answer a desired question is not particularly useful.

The importance of randomization in deciding when an intervention is sufficiently science based to be brought to the public needs to be reconsidered, and some consensus should be reached. Randomization has proved to be extremely difficult to implement in behavioral MSEs because of practical issues and political resistance. Multiple techniques, such as covariance analysis, multilevel modeling, and propensity scores, have been and are being developed for equating comparison groups that were not produced by randomization and may not be equivalent. The study described by Rog and Randolph in Chapter Five and the services analyses conducted for the MSE described by Cook and others in Chapter Three employed methods of this type. In deciding whether an intervention should be brought to the public, if no evidence from randomized studies is available, should evidence from MSEs based on such designs and analyses be considered sufficient? If findings from randomized trials and multisite studies with quasi-experimental studies exist, how should the two types of evidence be weighted?

Unpacking the Black Box. Methods for investigating the active ingredients in programs were not employed in all MSEs. Thus, interventions were sometimes operationally defined by a program label, with no consensus about how to go beyond the "black box" approach and investigate the effects of specific ingredients. Nevertheless, understanding the effects of specific ingredients is crucial to replicating programs and holds the possibility of identifying key changes that providers can make instead of adopting entire program models (see Chapter Five).

One approach for dealing with this issue is to specify the ingredients of all interventions in manuals generated in an intervention development phase preceding intervention testing. All therapists then receive comparable training and supervision in the manual-guided treatment. This approach, which is designed to guide intervention contents and ensure that interventions are implemented in a uniform way across all sites, is illustrated in the Marijuana Treatment Project MSE (see Chapter Two) and the Methamphetamine Treatment Project study (see Chapter Six).

In MSEs where there was less clarity about the components of specific interventions, investigators used several different approaches to try to unbundle intervention elements after the fact. Cook and others (in Chapter Three) measured the types and amounts of services that consumers received in different employment interventions and developed a cross-program measure to assess the presence or absence of program elements that were hypothesized as being crucial. Banks and others (Chapter Four) used expert judgment to differentiate programs, and Rog and Randolph (Chapter Five) developed fidelity measures that were implemented after the selection of programs. All of these approaches involve the use of statistical models to equate and compare individuals who are exposed to different program ingredients, as opposed to randomly assigning persons to these ingredients. The extent to which these models provide evidence that is definitive in nature is an important issue that remains to be resolved.

Dealing with Protocol Violations. Protocol violations occur when investigators cannot follow the design elements set in advance for the conduct of studies. Rog and Randolph (Chapter Five), for example, state that in some of their sites, randomized studies were initially proposed but were not implemented. Such protocol violations on the part of one or several sites in an MSE can potentially bias results, put study participants at risk, and even make studies nonviable. Principal investigators and project officers, in their zeal to complete studies, may not fully appreciate these risks.

The U.S. Food and Drug Administration (FDA) uses data safety monitoring boards to assess the degree to which studies have been compromised or changed by protocol violations and to determine whether subjects may have been put at risk. These boards are independent groups convened by the FDA and consist of persons who have no interest in the studies under review. The scientific advisory board convened for the Methamphetamine Treatment Project, described in Chapter Six, illustrates a step in this direction, although this board is described as influencing primarily the initial design of the study. At least one Substance Abuse and Mental Health Services Administration MSE steering committee (not described in this volume) voluntarily requested such an independent review when randomization procedures broke down. Data safety boards are neither required nor routinely used in MSEs of behavioral interventions. However, their use should be considered when protocol violations occur.

Producing Timely Findings. One reason for conducting MSEs is to obtain needed sample sizes more quickly in the interest of bringing interventions to the public (see Chapter One). However, other aspects of MSEs, including the use of lengthy consensus-building processes during the design phase, can delay the reporting of results (as noted in Chapter Three).

If MSEs are to speed up the process of bringing interventions to the public, mechanisms must be developed for producing interim findings that avoid breaking study blinds or otherwise biasing final study results. One way to do this would be to establish early data analysis groups that are separate from those responsible for conducting studies and preparing final reports of study results. These early data analysis groups would have to develop guidelines for qualifying their findings, since these findings would be based on partial and preliminary, not complete and final, data analyses. Such early analysis groups could also serve the function of monitoring subject safety, withdrawing persons from the study who met criteria for deterioration (see Chapter Two), or even terminating studies if substantial numbers of persons were deteriorating unexpectedly.

With respect to this challenge, the FDA Center for Drug Evaluation and Research (CDER) has developed review processes to speed the delivery of new drugs to consumers. These include standardized policies and improved communications designed to speed up the development of new products (Center for Drug Evaluation and Research, 1999). Similar innovations could be applied in MSEs.

Identifying Statistical Models for Analyzing Data from MSEs. Multisite studies by definition involve different geographical locations or, more generically, contexts (Chapter One, this volume). In addition to site-level context differences, target populations can also differ among sites and between conditions within sites (Chapter Four, this volume). There is currently little agreement regarding the best statistical models for analyzing multisite and repeated measures data (Chapter Four, this volume).

Several statistical approaches have been advanced to address these questions, including multilevel models (hierarchical linear models and other mixed-effects regression approaches) and prospective, meta-analytic approaches (Leff and others, 2002; Chapter Four, this volume).

As we learn more about the characteristics of behavioral interventions, it has become clear that in many multisite studies, the way in which specific intervention types are implemented tends to differ from one site to another, in much the same way that individuals randomly selected from populations differ from each other (Chapter Five, this volume). This suggests the suitability of random effects models in combining site data from multisite studies. However, we do not yet fully understand the advantages and disadvantages of the various approaches. It is hoped that our understanding will be increased through direct comparisons in parametric studies (Chapter Four, this volume).

A second analytic issue is the degree to which meta-analytic methods should be considered as a way to analyze data from MSEs themselves and to combine MSE findings with findings from other studies. Given the time and expense in testing behavioral interventions, consideration should be given to refining analytic techniques that make use of all available evidence. Synthesizing all available data contributes to bringing interventions to the public in a number of ways. First, combining the findings of MSEs with those of other studies gives a picture of which phases in the development of an intervention have been completed and which remain to be addressed. Also, although MSEs involve more programs and more varied consumers than single-site studies, combining MSE and other data may increase the number of programs and persons in subgroups, providing statistical power to investigate program level and subgroup effects (Chapter Four, this volume). Second, consensus about the utility of meta-analytic approaches might foster uniformity in how study results should be described in reports or published articles to make it possible to synthesize study results at a later date (Leff and others, 2002).

The Participatory Principle

The participatory principle implies that stakeholder groups should have meaningful input in all phases of MSEs. Stakeholders may include evaluators themselves, as well as government program and project officers, consumers of services, family members, and policymakers. All of the multisite studies examined in this volume had steering committees. These committees often consisted of evaluation scientists, consumers, and service developers and administrators (such as representatives from state mental health authorities), as well as government project officers. EIDP also convened a consumer assembly of from eight to fifteen consumers (Chapter Three, this volume). Without exception, these forums for stakeholder participation were viewed positively. However, some multisite investigators also noted several drawbacks.

On the positive side, multisite investigators mentioned the participatory processes as contributing to the values base (Chapter Two, this volume) and the scientific quality of studies (Chapter Five, this volume). Rog and Randolph (Chapter Five, this volume), for example, view the participatory process as creating an "invisible college" (Boruch and others, 1991) in which participants share knowledge and expertise.

On the negative side, the participatory process is described as being inefficient and time-consuming (Chapters Three and Five, this volume). In addition, it is seen as sometimes leading to decisions in which the methods chosen are driven by the capacities of the least capable sites (Chapter Five, this volume). Better site selection and study planning can address these issues.

Although all MSEs discussed the role of stakeholders on steering committees, there was little discussion of the roles of stakeholders in selecting topics for MSEs, developing Guidance for Applicants (GFA), and reviewing proposals. These roles are critical, since they define the boundaries and constraints within which studies must operate. More discussion of the positive and negative consequences of stakeholder participation in these processes and how to maximize the former and limit the latter is needed. The question raised by the participatory principle is this: When stakeholders other than evaluation scientists and funders collaborate on multisite projects, how should the interests and values of stakeholders be combined with the requirements of the science-based principle? Some issues related to the participatory principle follow.

Clarifying Stakeholder Roles in Designing the General Format of MSEs. With few exceptions, the funding agencies' prescriptiveness about the general format of multisite studies has been quite limited. In part, this results from funders' desire to allow investigators to add value through a study development process that takes advantage of the knowledge and experience of participating investigators and other stakeholders. GFAs typically specify the structure of the desired study in only the most general way. Furthermore, review panels are instructed to score applications on the basis of criteria such as scientific rigor, inclusiveness, and background of the investigators. These are all worthy criteria. However, they do not guarantee that the sites selected will fill an interesting policy space, nor do they ensure that the group of sites will even provide relevant comparisons. Furthermore, the absence of clearly defined minimum standards in most GFAs, with respect to those multisite design aspects that are critical, leaves open the possibility that sites not capable of complying with critical design elements will be funded. Finally, the fact that major aspects of the multisite design become clear only through a consensus process after sites are funded may place some sites in a difficult position with respect to local agreements that were obtained during the proposal preparation stage.

These weaknesses could be minimized if crucial aspects of study designs were specified more clearly in the GFA. The elements might include design features that are considered to be so important that they constitute minimal requirements for applicants. These features might include the following: (1) specification of the index intervention that explicitly defines crucial active ingredients, (2) equally explicit specification of what constitutes an acceptable comparison intervention, (3) specification of sampling procedures that might be considered crucial, and (4) specification of the databases to which investigators would be required to have access, such as Medicaid, block grant, or program databases.

Clarifying Stakeholder Roles in Defining Outcomes. Stakeholders should play a major role in defining outcomes. Consumers especially should be influential in deciding what constitutes effectiveness. The current debate over whether certain practices can be science based if they have not been shown to cause recovery, as designed by consumers, illustrates what can occur if consumers do not play a major role in choosing outcomes. The debate over whether science-based practices apply to certain racial, ethnic, and cultural groups also illustrates what happens when some groups feel excluded from the process of bringing interventions to the public.

Because different stakeholders are interested in different outcomes, when stakeholders play a major role in defining outcomes, MSEs may have the problem of addressing outcomes that they do not have the statistical power to investigate. To some extent, this appears to have happened in the MSEs described by Rog and Randolph in Chapter Five and Cook and others in Chapter Three. The supported housing MSE, for example, addressed a number of issues of importance to a variety of stakeholders: residential stability, level of functioning, satisfaction with housing, quality of life, and empowerment. Although a multistakeholder participatory process is admirable in its inclusiveness, the number and variety of outcomes are technically problematic. It is very difficult for even a multisite study to have sufficient statistical power to address a large number of diverse outcome variables. Part of the work in the development phase of an intervention might be to shorten the list of outcome variables as much as possible. Prior to any test of efficacy or effectiveness or comparison studies, a power analysis for each outcome variable might be desirable. In general, when multisite studies have a large number of diverse outcome variables, data reduction should be undertaken, and null findings should be treated with caution, given the possibility of underpowered statistical tests (Leff and others, 2002).

Clarifying Stakeholder Roles in Defining Safety. Stakeholders should also play a role in determining what constitutes safety and, conversely, what constitutes adverse events. The current debate over what constitutes coercion and whether programs of assertive community treatment are coercive illustrates what can occur if consumers do not play a major role in determining what constitutes an adverse event (Gomory, 1999). Nevertheless, debates over highly charged topics like coercion are difficult and time-consuming. New methods, such as the use of listserv discussions and mediation to reach consensus, coupled with the education of participants about issues related to timeliness, may be useful in this area. EIDP's several approaches to consumer involvement, including its listserv and consumer assembly, illustrate steps in the direction of involving stakeholders in MSEs in novel ways (see Chapter Three, this volume).

Clarifying Stakeholder Roles in Selecting Interventions for Testing. Stake-holders should be able to influence which interventions are tested, and they should be given the information to determine whether the tests are fair. The assertions by certain providers and consumers that their interventions were not given a chance to prove themselves or were held to different standards of proof from others illustrate what can happen if there is not equal access among stakeholder groups to the process of bringing interventions to the public (Dumont and Jones, forthcoming; Hogan, Roth, Svendsen, and Rubin, forthcoming). This problem might be ameliorated if stakeholders were given more access to the process of selecting interventions for testing and if consensus were reached on a set of steps for interventions to follow to be considered as proven safe and effective.

Reconciliation of the Scientific and Participatory Principles

The science-based and participatory principles present challenges to the evaluation of behavioral interventions. Combining the two in the design and execution of MSEs will inevitably create tensions. Science demands a sustained, deliberate approach to the accumulation of evidence. Consumers and providers, however, are eager for new and promising interventions to be offered to the public. Broad participation in the design of MSEs adds value by opening the process to diverse views. However, consensus-building processes have their price and may slow the evidence-building process.

Even as the challenges posed by the science-based and participatory principles are addressed, we should not expect that the process of bringing interventions to the public will be easy. Different stakeholders have different interests and values. Science-based knowledge will not necessarily resolve these differences. Moreover, even experimental evidence is subject to different interpretations.

At its core, the process of bringing an intervention to the public is in some part a matter of social conflict and construction (Bell, 1998). This is why the FDA's CDER process involves consensus panels, outside experts, and lawyers. However, having an explicit idea of a process that is accessible to stakeholders will facilitate the mediation and compromise that most processes will require. As Straw and Herrell suggest in Chapter One, this may result in the creation of learning communities to enhance cross-fertilization of ideas and to build evaluation and other capacity in local communities.

The thrust of this chapter (and this entire volume) is that a more systematic approach is needed for deciding when and how to conduct MSEs, when and how to analyze and report data, and when and how to involve nonevaluator stakeholders. This systematization will not happen if organizations (governmental, professional, scientific, advocacy, and so forth) do not take responsibility for monitoring and informing the process. Developing and adhering to such an approach will require resources and impose constraints on the evaluation process. To paraphrase Straw and Herrell in Chapter One, an important question to be addressed is this: If these constraints are not developed and followed, to what extent can we assert that we are bringing science-based interventions to the public?

Note

1. The idea that there should be an organization that guides the process of bringing behavioral interventions to the public is not a recent one. Rotter (1971) proposed this in 1971, and Godfried (1999) states that in 1980, Morris Parloff, a National Institute of Mental Health (NIMH) staff member, was called before a congressional committee in which he was asked if NIMH might function much like the U.S. Food and Drug Administration and specify which behavioral interventions were safe and effective.

References

Anthony, W. "The Need for Recovery-Compatible Evidence-Based Practices." *Mental Health Weekly,* 2001, 5(11), 5.

Bell, S. "Technology Assessment, Outcomes Data, and Social Context: The Case of Hormone Therapy." In P. Boyle (Ed.), *Getting Doctors to Listen: Ethics and Outcomes Data in Context.* Washington, D.C.: Georgetown University Press, 1998.

Bernal, G., and Scharro-del-Rio, M. "Are Empirically Supported Treatments Valid for Ethnic Minorities? Toward an Alternative Approach for Treatment Research." *Cultural Diversity and Ethnic Minority Psychology,* 2001, 7, 328–342.

Boruch, R., and others. "Sharing Confidential and Sensitive Data." In J. E. Sieber (Ed.), *Sharing Social Science Data: Advantages and Challenges.* Thousand Oaks, Calif.: Sage, 1991.

Center for Drug Evaluation and Research. *From Test Tube to Patient: Improving Health Through Human Drugs.* Rockville, Md.: U.S. Food and Drug Administration, 1999. [www.fda.gov/cder/about/whatwedo/testtube.pdf].

Dumont, J., and Jones, K. "Findings from a Consumer/Survivor Defined Alternative to Psychiatric Hospitalization." *Outlook,* forthcoming.

Godfried, M. "The Pursuit of Consensus in Psychotherapy Research and Practice." *Clinical Psychology: Science and Practice,* 1999, 6, 462–466.

Gomory, T. "Programs of Assertive Community Treatment (PACT): A Critical Review." *Ethical Human Sciences and Services,* 1999, 1(2), 1–17.

Hogan, M., Roth, D., Svendsen, D., and Rubin, B. "Transforming Research into Practice in a State Mental Health System." *Outlook,* forthcoming.

Leff, H. S., and others. "Knowledge Assessment: A Missing Link Between Knowledge Development and Application." Unpublished manuscript, 2002.

Newman, S. J. "Housing Attributes and Serious Mental Illness: Implications for Research and Practice." *Psychiatric Services,* 2001, 52, 1309–1317.

Rotter, J. "On the Evaluation of Methods of Intervening in Other People's Lives." *Clinical Psychologist,* Spring 1971, pp. 1–2.

H. STEPHEN LEFF *is director of the Evaluation Center at the Human Services Research Institute, Cambridge, Massachusetts.*

VIRGINIA MULKERN *is associate director of the Evaluation Center at the Human Services Research Institute, Cambridge, Massachusetts.*

INDEX

Back Issue/Subscription Order Form

Copy or detach and send to:
Jossey-Bass, 989 Market Street, San Francisco CA 94103-1741

Call or fax toll free!
Phone 888-378-2537 6AM-5PM PST; Fax 888-481-2665

Back issues: Please send me the following issues at $27 each.
(Important: please include series initials and issue number, such as EV77.)

1. EV _____

_____

_____

$ _____ Total for single issues

$ _____ SHIPPING CHARGES:

	SURFACE	Domestic	Canadian
First Item		$5.00	$6.50
Each Add'l Item		$3.00	$3.00

For next-day and second-day delivery rates, call the number listed above.

Subscriptions   Please ❑ start ❑ renew my subscription to *New Directions for Evaluation* for the year ____ at the following rate:

U.S.	❑ Individual $69	❑ Institutional $145
Canada	❑ Individual $69	❑ Institutional $185
All Others	❑ Individual $93	❑ Institutional $219

$ _____ Total single issues and subscriptions (Add appropriate sales tax for your state for single issue orders. No sales tax for U.S. subscriptions.Canadian residents, add GST for subscriptions and single issues.)

❑ Payment enclosed (U.S. check or money order only.)

❑ VISA, MC, AmEx, Discover Card #_____ Exp. date_____

Signature _____ Day phone _____

❑ Bill me (U.S. institutional orders only. Purchase order required.)

Purchase order #_____

Name _____

Address _____

Phone_____ E-mail _____

For more information about Jossey-Bass, visit our Web site at:
www.josseybass.com   **PRIORITY CODE = ND1**